The
Nuts & sprouts of
Healthy Eating

The Nuts & sprouts of Healthy Eating

Simple Steps to Eating Healthy and Losing Weight for Good

GAEL D. MEYER

FIRST EDITION · September 2011

15 14 13 12 11   5 4 3 2 1

ISBN 13: 978-0-9821405-7-4

Library of Congress: 2011938613

Manufactured in the United States of America.
Designed by James Monroe Design, LLC.

For information about special purchases or custom editions, please contact:

James Monroe Publishing, LLC.
A Division of James Monroe Design, LLC.
7236 Bald Eagle Lane
Willow River, Minnesota 55795

www.jamesmonroedesign.com

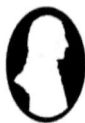

I would like to dedicate this book to my son Michael Rowan Meyer, an aspiring actor and writer so full of talent. His writing has inspired me to get my words out on paper and to help other people make the most of their lives by sharing the importance of healthy eating through organic foods.

DISCLAIMER

All of my recommendations and charts are general guidelines and meant to help you. There are always exceptions. I am not a doctor, and claim no absolute expertise or authority on health and wellness topics. This book is meant to be informative only, and is not a substitute for official medical advice.

CONTENTS

CONTENTS

ACKNOWLEDGMENTS

I would like to thank Anna and Kristen from Revitalive Health and Wellness Center in Newburyport, Massachusetts, for helping me get healthy again by showing me all about raw food eating. It has changed my life forever!

I would like to thank my niece, Sadie Dayton, with Sadie@SadiePhotography.com for helping with my photography in the book. She was a tremendous help and an excellent photographer!

I would like to thank Rita Barry-Corke from RBC Communications, and her talented husband, Mark, for a wonderful job with the video on my web site. I feel blessed to have found you and consider you both friends forever.

My editor Amy Quale has been great bringing me through my first book. She has done a wonderful job teaching and educating me through the process.

I would also like to thank Steve Harrison and the group of experts he has introduced me to over the past year through the Quantum Leap Program. Without his program I would not have this book; I would also have never learned so much about writing and marketing, nor the multitude of close-knit friends from the Q&L group whom I will be close with for years to come.

I want to say a big thank you to James Monroe from James Monroe Design for designing my first book and putting the group together to complete the publishing of my book! James was wonderful through this process, took all of my questions away, and was always there for me every step of the way!

I would like to extend a special thanks to Trey, for being such a good friend and someone who is always there for me and giving me good advice. You have always believed in me even when I didn't!

Thanks to Jay Forte, who has entered my life over the past year and became a great friend and confidant. Thank you so much for bouncing ideas back and forth and keeping me positive at all times!

A special thanks to Wendy Lipton-Dibner, who recently entered my life as my new Mastermind Coach for the year. Wendy is extraordinary in her teachings and presence on stage. I know I will benefit tremendously over the next year from her gifted talents.

MISSION

My mission is to help people realize the importance of eating healthy, organic, whole foods, and show others how health is directly related to what we eat! I will also show how to make changes to a current way of eating that will have a positive impact on health and weight.

It is time for each of us to take responsibility for our own health, and to question traditional medicine on almost every level before assuming it is the only choice. It is my hope in the future years to be able to help fund a completely alternative health clinic for people interested in healing themselves naturally without drugs.

"LET FOOD BE YOUR MEDICINE
AND MEDICINE BE YOUR FOOD"

—*Hippocrates*

INTRODUCTION

Does it seem like every time you look around someone is going on or off a diet, trying to find that quick
fix for weight loss and perfect health? There are many
people struggling with the issues of losing weight
and getting healthy in today's society. The average
American is overweight by anywhere from twenty
to one hundred pounds, so if you could stand to lose
a few, you are not alone out there. I was once there
myself. I tried all kinds of diets growing up, only to
end up gaining more weight back, weighing more
than when I started. Do you ever wonder why most
other cultures seem to be in better shape than we
are in the United States? What is it that has so many
Americans out of shape these days?

Weight and overall health is subjective, but it's
safe to say the convenience of bad foods contributes
greatly to our society's poor health. Everywhere we
look, we see fast food restaurants making it convenient, easy, and cheap to eat bad foods. How did this
happen? Well, our fast-paced way of living has changed
our culture over the years. Our mindset has become
the problem and our food has become the byproduct

of this problem. Our culture has become so busy that we are working more hours. Smart phones, tablets, and computers have sped up our lives, allowing us to do more in a day than we ever thought possible. So how do we work all of these hours and have time to eat? We chow down on on-the-run foods, making us the prime target for antacids and upset stomachs. This is where the industry has kicked in for our convenience and, because fast food is so inexpensive, people tend to get twice as much food than they actually need. Still, even eating twice the food doesn't seem to make us full. This is because most of the fiber has been ripped out of our food; through processing and added sugar, not only is this food triggering us to eat more instead of less, but it isn't making us full!

These foods draw us in with their smell, taste, appearance, price, and their convenience to our lives. People are always in a hurry, wanting things immediately; unfortunately, our health has suffered for it. We have gotten away from making our meals from scratch and sitting down together in an unhurried environment with our friends and family.

When I was younger, there weren't any fast food places around, so I ate at home or packed my own meals. Now convenience has taken over our lives; this is a big downfall of our society today and a large contributing factor to our poor health and obesity as a society.

This book can benefit any style eater, whether you are a meat eater, vegetarian, vegan, or a raw vegan like me. I have been each of these at one time or another in my life. Everyone has their own preferences as to what they wish to eat; in this book, I will help you make better choices, additions, or alterations to whichever way you choose to eat.

I will also show you how you can comfortably eat out in restaurants, others' homes, and how to enjoy holiday meals without feeling separate from everyone else. As long as you eat well most of the time, there is no need to beat yourself up because you make different choices at particular times. Your body is very forgiving. Give yourself permission to make different choices occasionally.

I hope you find this book helpful and informative, easily showing how you can make some changes a little at a time and create better health (and weight loss, if you choose) for you and your family.

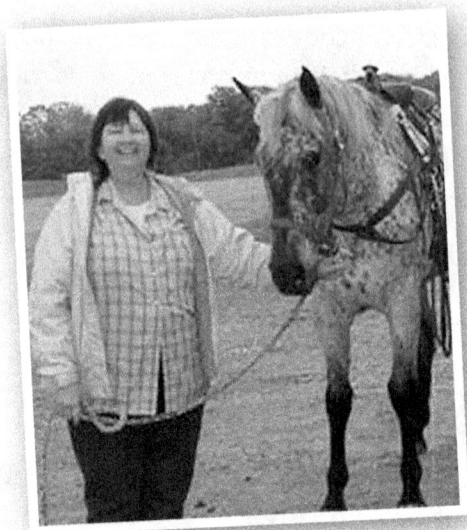

BEFORE

AFTER

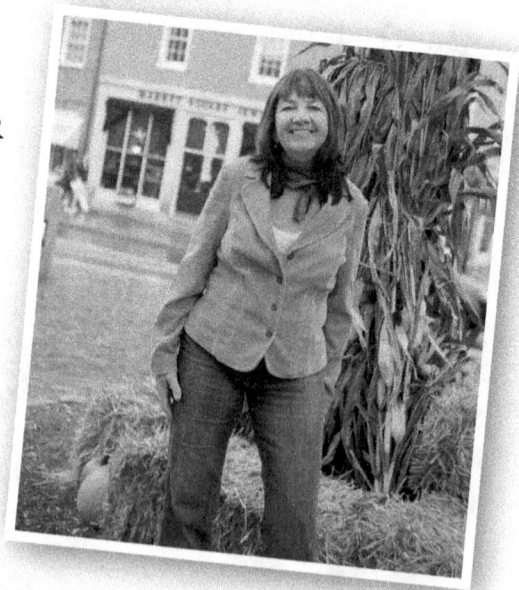

MY STORY

I grew up in a large family of seven brothers and sisters in Topsfield, Massachusetts. Things were pretty strict in my family. When dinnertime came, we weren't allowed to leave the table until everything was off of our plates. Unfortunately, we didn't have a dog to help us out under the table. My mother was a great cook, and so eating a lot was never difficult! My favorite meals were on Sundays. She would typically cook a roast beef, chicken, turkey, or pork chops. On Fridays we always had fish. My mother could make the best baked haddock ever. I still can taste it just thinking about it. She rarely bought any food out of a box, which unfortunately is the way of life these days. We had our milk delivered by a milk man in glass bottles, eggs from a local farmer, and fresh veggies. Most of the chicken and meat came from free-range sources.

Cooking back then was a process that took time, especially with our large family of nine, and involved everyone helping out. The food was much healthier than most foods nowadays, and tasted better too; there were no chemicals, preservatives, and very little processed food. There were no instant mashed potatoes boxes, premade store-bought meals, or microwave ovens in our family. Everything was from scratch. Our food was from whole grains, fresh veggies and fruit, and all organic. The soil was much better back when I was growing up because there were fewer chemicals, additives, and genetic modifications of foods in the farming industry. Preparing the meal and eating would bring my family together, and mealtime was a time for us to talk about the things we did that day. Sunday was the really special big meal day and we all looked forward to the smells, taste, and being with our family.

Growing up, I was kind of chubby; this was mostly due to a sedentary life and eating too much bread and desserts. I grew up in the country so there were things to do outside, but it just wasn't my thing when I was a kid, though that changed as I got older.

When I was about twelve, I joined the 4-H Club and started taking care of a neighbor's horse. I loved this very much. I would go out for long rides through the woods. I then started ice skating on the local pond about half a mile from my house, and went for long walks exploring the woods and looking for animals. I also remember spending hours in the tree in front of my house watching newborn baby birds being born and taking notes about how they grew up. I was getting a lot more exercise and started slimming down some.

As I became a teenager, boys started to interest

me, so I went on all kinds of diets to get into better shape. I remember my mother putting me on a diet where I nearly starved myself. It consisted of cottage cheese, carrots, celery, water, a piece of baked chicken and veggies for dinner, and no snacks at all—just so I could fit into a dress I wanted to wear for the school dance. At the same time, I joined softball and gymnastics teams at school. I remember being so hungry, especially with all of the new activities I was doing. All I can remember thinking about was FOOD! I had the most intense cravings for bread, butter, desserts, and Sunday morning doughnuts. I did lose weight and get in shape, but it wasn't a pleasant experience. I always seemed to stay around sizes ten and twelve. I looked good, but not as thin as my friends. It seemed like most of my life had been consumed with losing weight, getting into shape, and thinking about food—a perpetual merry-go-round.

Then I was off to college in Boston, right in time for the hippie generation. I was totally into that. I didn't do any hardcore drugs, but I did sample a bit. Dorm food was hugely fattening and full of breads, gravy, and desserts. Speed was the crave in all of the dorms back then for anyone looking to lose weight or stay up all night cramming for tests, so I was all over that. I remember losing weight because of this and balancing school and as much fun and extracurricular activities I could manage. All that to get down to a solid size nine! Unfortunately, there are always consequences for bad behavior. I got sick from not eating or sleeping enough. That laid me up for two weeks. And of course I gained all the weight back. It did teach me a lesson, though.

After school, I met a musician and took off with him and his band for a couple of years. That was a life of long hours and really bad, calorie-packed diner food. I always had to take a nap after eating out this way. That was very challenging for me. After traveling around with him for a year or two, we parted ways and I headed back east to Topsfield where I grew up.

Shortly after that, I met someone else and we moved up to Barrington, New Hampshire. My boy-friend and I moved into a big house that we shared with a bunch of other people who were also very earthy and healthy. They taught me all about how to be a vegetarian. At the age of twenty-one, I became a vegetarian. Using this eating lifestyle, it was easier for me to maintain my weight and keep healthy. I had had a hard time maintaining my weight in the past if I was not active, but eating right and getting a lot of exercise outside kept me active and trim.

I loved this way of eating, and started making my own yogurt, maple syrup, and growing my own vegetables. I even started grinding my own berries into flour and making my own bread. I started mak-ing all of my meals from scratch (kind of like my mom used to do!). Eating consisted of rice and vegeta-bles and salads every day. In the beginning I was hun-gry about every three to four hours and I thought I was going to start gaining weight again, but I didn't.

The food was fresh, whole, and full of good fiber. One thing I learned was that the more bread I ate, the quicker I gained weight. So I kept my bread intake to a minimum. I listened to my body and ate when I was hungry, just not a lot at any one time.

I met my lifelong best friends, Don and Leslie, while I was in Barrington. They lived in a teepee about half a mile from our house, which was right next to a beautiful river. I loved it there and we all quickly became fast friends and still are today. Soon after, I got teepee as well, and lived across the street and up a hill from Don and Leslie.

I broke up with my boyfriend before moving into the teepee with my dog Tara. I loved this life which was so full of life and nature! My kitchen was set up outside where I stored my seeds, nuts, and grains in glass jars. I had cast-iron skillets and a stove that went over the fire pit to cook with. Don, Leslie, and I shared a huge garden with lots of fresh vegetables to eat. I would walk, ride my bike, and hike a lot. We all took up meditation and did the whole spiritual-lifestyle thing. Life was good. My friends eventually had to move to Wyoming for work. I kept up with the vegetarian lifestyle for many years to come.

About three years later, while I was in my mid-twenties, I met some people who were teaching nutrition. I loved this and found it totally fascinating. I took a couple of classes and was going to jump right into this as a profession, but I got sidetracked (which happened often in my life). I met another man and moved in with him and his two children, whom I am still very close with today. I remember turning them all into vegetarians. Oh, how they must have hated me at the time. They were young and so used to eating junk food and sweets. They both actually eat very healthy today, though.

We parted ways after about seven years and I went out west to Laramie, Wyoming to visit my best friends. I loved it out there so much that I decided to move there, and ended up staying for about twelve years. I bartended at the Cowboy Bar in Laramie. That was a trip. I didn't even like country music when I moved out there, but it grew on me. I got my first horse there. His name was Medicine. I would always be out hiking, horseback riding, camping, and rock climbing and skiing. About two years after getting Medicine, I went horse packing in the mountains for three months. While on this trip, I brought brown rice, dehydrated vegetables and fruit, and a fishing pole. As I was limited in food I could eat on this trip, I decided to occasionally eat fish because I knew it was very fresh and coming from crystal-clean waters, though for the most part I did not eat fish. I was very healthy and thin on that trip with all of the exercise up and down mountains with my horses. I remained a vegetarian here, even in meat country.

A few years later I took a trip to Israel for three months and lived in a Kibbutz. I know, I was all over the place with my life—but I was footloose and fancy free! My time in Kibbutz was a wonderful experience, and the reason I am bringing it up is because I wanted to share the eating lifestyle of the people in Israel. They are the most beautiful, physically fit people I have ever come across. They do a lot of walking, and eat very well. There would be salads for breakfast, which took some getting used to, lots of fruit, vegetables, and water. Lunch was their main meal of the day, which consisted of beans and rice, and dinner was a light meal of salads and fruit. When I went into the city you didn't see McDonald's restaurants. What you did see were lots of stands selling falafels or organic rice and bean wraps. There was no junk food anywhere. I am sure things have changed since I was there, but I was very impressed.

While I was in Wyoming I met someone else, and together we moved to Missouri. That was a big mistake, but I was stuck there for a while. We got married and divorced in the course of a year, and I had to stick around because I had little money. A couple of years later, I met another man and fell in love. I married this man and had my son Michael, the love of my life, at the age of thirty-five. I was still a vegetarian, but my husband ate meat and dairy, drank, and smoked cigarettes. I should have realized right then that it would never work! I got divorced again, moved back east, and stayed with my parents until I found my own place.

This was the first time in my life that I had responsibilities. I had a son to raise and care for on my own, which required money of course. So, I got my real estate license and have been in real estate for almost three decades now.

It didn't take me long to get back into shape, as I was eating healthy and remained active. I took up tennis and was out hiking with my son every chance I had. I was in the best shape I had been in for a long while. When my son was about eight years old, I decided to take a self-defense class which was being offered at the same place my son was taking karate lessons. On the last day of this class, something went terribly wrong. I was throwing a 250-pound man over my shoulder under the supervision of the teacher. Unfortunately, the teacher was not watching very carefully. I had the wrong leg out, and consequently the man landed on my left leg—fracturing my tibia in three places. The whole class cheered so loud that they did not realize I was actually screaming from excruciating pain. The teacher then came over and looked at my leg, and decided he would straighten it; this caused further breakage and pain.

This was not a happy time in my life. I was in the hospital for ten days. I actually died twice on the table, and thankfully was able to be brought back. I had no insurance, nor did the karate establishment. My wonderful, happy life suddenly disappeared in a blink. Here I was, on my own, raising my son by myself, and no longer able to work. The money I had just saved up for our first house went to medical bills.

After about six months, I could go out with crutches with a brace on my leg. I could not walk very fast or far, and had a difficult time navigating stairs, which kept me from going back to work at that time. I couldn't get around, drive, or go upstairs—as these are all necessary abilities for a real-estate agent, I was out of work for about nine months. After depleting my funds down to twenty-five cents in my pocket, I went on welfare so I could get insurance and food for my son. I was on crutches for a total of two years. This was also very hard on my young son at the time. I couldn't even tuck him into bed anymore, nor could I go out and play with him.

I went from being an active, healthy person to a couch potato in one day. I started gaining around ten pounds a year. Being on welfare, my meals were minimal. I had to buy the cheapest and most filling food so we would have enough to eat every week. That consisted of white bread, milk, cheap soups loaded with salt and preservatives, cheese that was meant to last for ten years (wrong on so many levels!), and I got hooked on the old-time, fattening, processed foods and snacks.

I replaced my ability to exercise with my ability to eat junk food. Food filled the void in my life, which of course only made me more depressed. I would lose some weight only to gain more back. I am sure many of you have been through that rat race. I could no longer do any of the activities I loved that kept me in shape, so I went from diet to diet only for them all to fail. I tried the liquid diets, high-protein diets, and the carbohydrate diets. Heck, I even tried the diets that deliver the meals directly to your house. None of them worked for very long. I would just gain everything back or more when the diet ended. That was my biggest mistake; I went on diets. Diets are meant to end, which is why they don't work. A person needs to change their diet forever—not go on a temporary diet.

I pushed myself deeper and deeper into work, trying to focus on making a better life for my son. I wanted to be able to send him to private high school so he could thrive and fulfill his dreams. I joined a coaching company for real estate, thinking that maybe this was the way to make a leap in my career. This ended up being a great decision. I started making a lot more money, and was able to send my son to private school where he graduated at the top of his class. I was doing so well that I bought a house in Gloucester, Massachusetts and tore it down and built my dream house on the water. I still live here and love it to this day. It is very peaceful and beautiful, with lots of birds all around me. I was also able to send my son to college. Things were good, at least in that part of my life.

I was really lucky to have such great clients during this tough time in my life. None of them treated me any differently when I gained my weight. I was good at my job, and they saw the fact that I truly cared about them and delivered what I said I would. Dating, however, was a different story. Mostly, I didn't feel like dating because I was still attracted to men who were outdoorsy, healthy, and fit. I was no longer any of those things. Men no longer looked at me like they used to. So I hung out with my friends or alone; I also spent more time with the new friends I added to my life: unhealthy snacks. I tried to fill the void I had with food. This did not work, however. My self-esteem was very low, although I did not show it to anyone else. I always had a smile on my face in public. I kept my feelings inside instead of sharing them, which would have been the best thing for me to do. Even though I had bounced back in so many ways, I was still embarrassed and ashamed of myself. I gave up hope.

Everything was great . . . except me! There was still something missing in my life: my health and the love of the outdoors that I always cherished so much. In 2007, I weighed eighty pounds more than I once weighed. I was obese! I really felt unhealthy, like I was sick from the inside now. Everything ached and hurt. I was sick all the time, my legs always hurt, my back was always going out, I had acid reflux, and I felt I was going in the direction of needing medical attention soon. I had no idea what I was going to do. I wanted to be there for my son growing up, and I was starting to wonder if I would be able to.

Then one day, my good friend Trey told me of some women who opened a health and wellness center in Newburyport, Massachusetts called Revitalive Health and Wellness Center. I decided that I had nothing to lose, so I went there. At that point in my life, I didn't go for weight loss like I had in the past. I went in to see if they could help me get healthy naturally. These women offered a whole new change in lifestyle for me, and I embraced this change. I had been a vegetarian since I was twenty-one, but this was something different. At their recommendation, I became a raw vegan. I combined that with a series of cleanses and colonic hydrotherapy.

I began to feel wonderful again and actually ate more food than I had ever eaten in my life. I no longer starved myself. I did everything they told me to do, and lost eighty pounds in a short eight months! All of my symptoms went away; my legs got better, I rarely got sick, and my acid reflux went away and never came back. I can now do all the things I used to do, such as hike, climb mountains, play tennis, and run. And, I look fifteen years younger! To date, I have not been sick for four years, and have kept the eighty pounds off . . . truly amazing!

My whole outlook on life changed. I now love getting up in the morning again. I love going for a walk every day, knowing that I won't feel fatigued or achy. I feel so healthy again, and my self esteem is back full force. All of my friends and coworkers compliment me, saying I look years younger. People ask me how I lost the weight and got healthy again. Hope and pride have reentered my life, and I can once again look myself in the mirror and smile. You can see my before and after pictures in this book. I can help you accomplish your goals too.

After four years of being a raw vegan, something extraordinary happened. I joined this incredible group called Quantum Leap, which is a group for writers who wish to make a difference in someone else's life. I had always dreamed about writing, but never thought I was good enough. I realized that a passion I had many years earlier in my life resurfaced: nutrition. Only this time, I combined my love for nutrition with a way that I can express and share it with others; by writing, speaking, and coaching about my experiences over these past four years (and really, all my years), I get to give hope to other people going through similar struggles.

MAKING POSITIVE CHANGES
IN EATING

I am not expecting everyone to embrace the raw vegan lifestyle. It was right for me. My goal is to try to help people become more aware of how they can actually heal themselves and lose weight by what they eat or don't eat—these ideas can work for vegetarians, vegans, raw vegans, or meat eaters. Everyone needs to take charge of their own health. Not the doctors, hospitals, family or friends—YOU! Doctors and hospitals have their places, but not necessarily in nutrition. That is up to each individual to learn and take charge of. I am here to show people how to get healthier naturally. Wouldn't it be wonderful if the choice to eat better alone could possibly dramatically improve your health, without medicines and surgeries? It certainly could not hurt you, and could only improve your health.

Recently, there have been more and more organic farms springing up all over the United States. This is proof that people are starting to see the correlation between organic eating and our health. I see the world changing back to this way of life . . . the way of our parents and their parents, when everyone ate more greens, and the soil was healthier. Most people do not understand the importance of eating certified organic fruits, veggies, and whole foods. There are huge differences between food that is organic and food that is not.

If your food is not organic, it most likely has chemicals and additives and could be genetically modified, which is not the way Mother Nature intended them to be. A good example of this is soy products. Unless you are getting organic soy beans, who knows what they really are? You won't be getting as many vitamins and minerals from food that is not organic because the soil is not as rich in nutrients, and a lot of food that is not organic is processed, stripping it of most of its nutrients and fiber. Organic food, on the other hand, is rich in vitamins, minerals, enzymes, and nutrients, and has no chemicals or additives. It is just natural, whole food. And it tastes better, too.

Eating nonorganic and processed foods is potentially a reason that so many people in the United States today are vitamin and mineral deficient, overweight, and sick. Instead of relying on organic healthy food to heal ourselves, we rely on medicines and drugs to make us feel better. We are not fixing and eliminating the problems; we are treating the symptoms, not the cause. We are in essence, just putting a Band-Aid on most of our problems. In some cases, we can actually make things worse by taking drugs and over-the-counter medicines. Just listen to the TV—when a new drug comes out, half of the commercial is telling all about the side effects. Staying healthy is very simple . . . most of it is just about what you eat.

WHY IS OUR NATION SO OVERWEIGHT AND UNHEALTHY?

Obesity is a very common problem in the United States. Currently, about a third of all Americans suffer from obesity. This in turn creates more sickness and disease and a lot more trips to the doctor's office, buying medicines and quick fixes, and the hospital.

A lot of people probably heard or saw President Clinton when he spoke about his health in 2010. He spoke about his battle with cholesterol, clogged arteries, and the bypass and stint he had to have implanted in his body. He was scheduled for another stint because the first one was short lived, but chose to seek out an alternative healing approach to his health with a plant-based diet with vegan and raw vegan food. He went off dairy and meat and chicken and basically ate beans, legumes, plants, vegetables, fruit, almond milk, and a protein supplement. With this eating lifestyle, President Clinton lost twenty-four pounds and his plaque buildup is gone. He looks and feels great, just from changing what he ate! Many diseases and medical problems can really be eliminated or changing the way we eat. President Clinton has named T. Colin Campbell, PhD and his son Thomas M. Campbell, II, MD [who co-authored *The China Study*] as a resource in his interview.

In *The China Study*, researchers explore how societies can be vastly different in health based on what they eat. Much of the research analyzes the way we eat in the United States, with far too much animal protein; the authors believe this is the reason for many diseases, including cancer. The author grew up on a dairy farm and changed his whole life after this research. He stopped eating meat and dairy after he found out how harmful it is to the body. "All animal protein, not just fatty meats, raises cholesterol levels . . ." says T. Colin Campbell.

Statistics Comparing Chinese and American Dietary Intakes

HealthyEatingHealthyBody@gmail.com

NUTRIENT	CHINA	US
Calories (kcal/kg body weight/day)	2,641	1,989
Total fat (% of calories)	14.5	34-38
Dietary Fiber (g/day)	33	12
Total Protein (g/day)	64	91
Animal Protein (% of total calories)	0.8	10-11
Total Iron (mg/day)	34	18

Campbell, T. Colin, PhD, Thomas M. Campbell II, MD.
The China Study. 74, Figure 4.3

Overeating the wrong foods and under activity, are the most common causes of weight gain. The modern diet today is high in fat, which has twice as many calories as proteins or carbohydrates do. Processing has removed low-calorie fiber and bulk from most foods, so what is left is unbalanced, condensed, and fattening foods, all leading to obesity.

We are not eating enough uncooked, unprocessed whole fruits, raw veggies, sprouts, greens, and whole-grain foods. Whole foods fill you up faster and stay with you longer. They are full of enzymes, vitamins, minerals, and fiber. The majority of calories you consume should come from raw foods which are low in fat and high in nutrition. This will help prevent overeating and will also provide the added benefit of additional vitamins, minerals, fiber, and enzymes. This is very important because enzymes are what breaks up the fat cells in your body and eliminates excess fat. Enzymes are found in raw, uncooked, organic foods.

It is a shame, but it is more expensive to eat healthy in this country. Whole foods are not promoted enough by our government to keep the prices down. This also goes for the organic free-range meat farms. Because it is less expensive to buy junk food and processed food, especially if you have a large family to feed, people end up eating all of the wrong types of food. They end up eating fattening, over-processed, low-fiber foods without enzymes, vitamins, or minerals. The lack of nutrients in these convenient foods makes the eater end up eating more to try to fill up, thus taking in more calories at one sitting than is good for you, without even realizing it. These bad foods are easily accessible and fast. People have to learn to make the time to make good food if they are ever going to get off of the merry-go-round of over-eating and being unhealthy.

WHAT WOULD DRIVE YOU
TO MAKE A HUGE CHANGE
IN YOUR LIFE?

Does Pleasure Drive You or
Does Pain Drive You?

Everyone is different. For me, it was pain that drove me to make a change for my health. I felt sick inside, and I could no longer walk more than ten minutes without having to rest. The fact that I wouldn't be around for my son if I didn't get healthy was another huge factor. *What is the point to my life if I cannot see him grow up and become the man he is to become?* I thought. Could I really live the rest of my life not doing the things I loved to do so much? I decided, based on these painful realizations that I could not, I WOULD not, let myself continue on my unhealthy path! I discovered that changing my diet changed everything in my life . . . and all for the better! My pain went away on so many levels, not just my physical pain, but my emotional pain as well.

Everyone who goes on a diet does it for a specific reason. Some want to lose weight, some want to feel better and improve their health. What drives you to make a big change in your life? What drives you? Pain or pleasure?

The pain you could experience by not eating well:

- allergies
- headaches
- fibromyalgia
- heart disease
- diabetes
- cancer
- premature wrinkles
- constipation diarrhea
- exhaustion
- insomnia
- ineffective immune system
- lethargy
- tumors
- gallstones

- lack of focus and concentration
- dry skin, brittle nails, dry hair, acne
- weight gain
- feeling judgment from others because of your weight

What pleasures would you experience if you were healthy again from eating well?

- fewer headaches
- less frequent flu or sickness
- fewer allergies
- weight loss
- looking good
- feeling good
- having tons of energy again
- having soft beautiful hair, hard nails, and smooth, clear skin
- Being able to sleep through the night
- potentially going off medications
- potentially reversing diabetes
- potentially reversing heart disease
- playing your favorite sport again

- having fun with children
- having your significant other look at you the way they used to
- having fun shopping again

The list can go on and on depending what you like. You need to decide which list you want to live in. The choice is yours, and it is mostly all about what you eat or are not eating that determines which list you will live with. Make the best choice for your life and health!

FIFTEEN FREQUENTLY-ASKED QUESTIONS AND ANSWERS

1) Q. Do I have to be a raw vegan, vegan, or vegetarian to lose weight and be healthy?

A. No you do not have to be, but if you can at least incorporate pieces of those eating styles, it can greatly benefit and speed things up in your mission to be healthy. For example, make sure you eat a lot more vegetables and fruits, both raw and blended (like in a smoothie). You could always start out being a vegetarian first and do it in steps. Try eliminating meat or dairy first for two weeks and see how you feel.

2) Q. Do I have to eat three meals a day and also snacks?

A. If you want to lose weight, not be hungry, and get rid of cravings, yes. I would at least try to do one to three snacks but only if you need the snacks. If you aren't hungry, don't eat the snacks. If you are working out a lot, it is important to add additional calories in the form of snacks. You should definitely eat three meals a day. I am not talking huge, must-take-a-nap-after-eating kinds of meals. Keep your evening meal lighter than your lunch if possible. If you skip meals your body shuts down so you actually are burning less calories and fat. If you're eating every three to four hours, your body is always working and your insulin levels should remain at a working level, which will keep you from being hungry all of the time and eating the wrong types of foods. You will find that if you don't wait until you are hungry to eat, you won't be starving or craving certain foods, especially if you are also drinking your eight glasses of water during the day.

3) Q. What if I eat something bad for me over the weekend?

A. Just pick up where you left off. If you do go out to eat or go to someone's home for dinner, just try to eat more vegetables, grains, legumes, and nuts, and try to skip the meat, bread, and desserts.

4) Q. Do I need to give up coffee and tea?

A. Well, everything in moderation is always a good thing, especially if you are trying to lose weight. A big reason people can't lose weight is because they get cravings from things that we get addicted to—caffeine is a huge culprit. Try using less coffee, and when you do have some, ask for organic coffee to avoid added chemicals. You could also opt for caffeine-free organic tea if your desire is to drink a hot liquid rather than to have caffeine.

5) Q. But I love dairy, especially cheese!

A. Cheese was the hardest to give up for me as well; it's so bad for you and your figure! Aside from being acidic, dairy is high in fat and calories, and can create a haven of food allergies in a lot of people and children. If you choose to eat cheese occasionally, eat organic free-range cheese or organic goat cheese, but do so sparingly. If you have a pizza, ask for goat cheese on the side (no other cheese) so you can put it on yourself, and ask for thin crust without meat. Just add sauce, herbs, and a lot of veggies. There is also non-dairy vegan cheese which melts down well. Most organic stores have this is the refrigerated section.

6) Q. Butter? But I love butter!

A. If you can't give up butter, make sure it comes from organic free-range cows and is real butter, not margarine or anything fat-free or diet. And, use it sparingly. You can also just use organic olive oil on your potato. If you eat fish, try just squeezing a lemon on it instead of adding the butter as well. You will be surprised how good it tastes just like that. So what are the differences between butter and margarine and why should you care?

Margarine: Margarine is made from vegetable oils. If you see the words "partially hydrogenated" in front of any vegetable oil, the food contains trans fats. (Note: most packages of margarine say that the product contains no trans fats—but partially hydrogenated oils ARE trans fats.) Eating hydrogenated fats has been linked diabetes and heart disease.

Butter: Butter comes from the fatty cream of cow's milk. There are differences between organic butter and non-organic butter. Organic butter has not been processed, and therefore all its nutrients or vitamins are intact. In non-organic butter, the milk or cream has been homogenized (ground into small particles so that the cream cannot rise to the top) and/or pasteurized (essentially, cooked), which means it has lost a good portion of its natural nutritional value. Non-organic butter could contain preservatives, which is great for shelf life but bad for your digestion. Preservatives inhibit food from going bad, but also inhibit your body's ability to break it down in order to obtain energy from it.

Organic butter is an excellent source for vitamin A (retinal), vitamin D, vitamin K, vitamin E, and protein. Vitamin A, when obtained from organic butter, absorbs very easily into your body. If you are lucky enough to have a source of butter from cows that only graze on green grass (free-range organic), you are in for consuming large amounts of vitamins. A, D, K, E, and protein are just a few to mention.

7) Q. What about bread?

A. If you want to lose weight, lose the bread or at least cut way down. When you do buy bread, try sprouted whole grain varieties in the freezer section. One brand I use when I have bread is called Ezequiel. They also make English muffins etc. There is also gluten-free bread called Mana in the freezer section. As healthy as these breads are, they still should be consumed sparingly. Nothing will put on weight faster than eating bread. When you make sandwiches, try using large leafs of lettuce instead of bread. You are saving a lot of unnecessary calories and fat that way, plus you are getting more greens and it crunches. The crunching of foods is very satisfying.

Have you ever taken a slice of white bread and rolled into a ball? It becomes very small and gooey. Take a piece of whole grain bread and put it next to the white bread. Most, if not all, of the fiber has been removed from the white bread, which is why most people will sit and eat two to four pieces of bread in one sitting. When you eat whole-grain bread it is so much more filling and takes longer to eat because it is full of fiber. The reason sprouted whole grain breads are better for you is that you are getting much more vitamins and minerals that are easier for your body to digest (because the grain berries have already sprouted).

When choosing a grain or bread, the top ingredients to look for are whole-sprouted wheat and organic-rolled oats. These should be the first ingredients in any grain product, including cereal.

8) Q. Won't I be hungry and bored eating vegetables, salads, and organic foods?

A. For me, it is quite the opposite. With the additional vegetables and greens you will be adding to your meals, you will feel more satisfied and full. There will be a lot of fiber in the salads and the whole-grain products you will substitute for the traditional over-the-counter packaged foods. Your salads can be a delightful and beautiful addition to your meals. They don't and shouldn't be boring. Use mixed greens, spinach, different colored vegetables including celery, carrots, peppers, and sprouts. Then add grapes or apples, some baby frozen peas, almonds or walnuts, and onions. Try topping it off with some fresh avocado. Then use organic salad dressing or olive oil. You don't have to put all of these things in one salad, and you can mix it up. It can be a beautiful creation which your family will look forward to eating. Bottom line: Because the foods you will be eating will be full of fiber and nutrients, and because they don't have added sugar that acts as triggers to eat more, you will naturally feel more satisfied.

9) Q. Is this a vegan diet?

A. I personally am a raw vegan, but you do not need to be. Again, just try to incorporate a lot of organic raw food with the way you currently eat. The more organic and raw vegetables and greens you can incorporate into your eating, the healthier you will become. You can always start out small and keep adding more of the good stuff. Remember you will have the benefit of getting important enzymes into your body from the raw food. So just add those to the rest of your meal, no matter what style you choose. Try cutting back on meat. If you can't give it up, start eating organic free-range meat and fish that does not come from a fishery. Eat the way you choose, but make a few healthy alterations to start.

10) Q. What about desserts?

A. Traditional desserts are full of sugar and calories, and make you hungry after you eat them because of the sugar spikes created in your blood. There are other things you can teach your body to like. You can offer fresh fruits as a dessert after your dinner has settled. Or you can make some of your favorite desserts but instead of using sugar when making your favorite dessert, use an alternative sweetener; in place of milk, use almond milk, or free-range organic whole milk; instead of white flour, use an organic flour; use organic fruits and real organic butter. This will cut back on the calories and fat content of your desserts.

Remember, if you eat fruit after your meal as a dessert, wait a while as fruits digest more quickly than heavier foods and you don't want it just sitting in your stomach and fermenting. I have a food combining chart in this book to show you how long certain foods take to digest. There is also raw chocolate out there now! It is much healthier for you, and you don't feel a need for lots of it like you would if you grabbed a regular candy bar off the shelf. It also does not give you a headache. They also make vegan and raw vegan deserts fresh in some of the organic restaurants. Yummy! You can also make a lot of vegan desserts including raw ice cream. I can't tell the difference. You should always try to cut back on too many desserts of course.

11) Q. But if I go off a lot of these foods, how will I get enough protein and vitamins?

A. There is a huge myth about how much protein we need in our diets, and the type of protein. The worst protein you can eat is from meat or meat products like dairy. Our bodies process meat differently than we process vegetables, turning a lot of it to sugar, which makes our bodies very acidic. If you eat a lot of organic foods and eat a lot of the veggies raw, you will be getting more than enough protein. For instance, spinach has more protein than steak. Even broccoli has more than steak, but it is an alkaline-based protein which is more easily assimilated in the body. Some good sources of protein are hemp seeds, chia seeds, spinach, nuts, and beans. There is a long list. For more information on vegetable-based protein, refer to *Healing Cancer from the Inside Out* and *The Rave Diet & Lifestyle* by Mike Anderson. The USDA dietary guidelines call for protein levels above 10 percent of total calories. Ten percent is four times what the average adult actually needs. This exaggeration unfortunately is based more on the needs of food lobbies selling high-protein foods rather than on human needs. You may think humans can never get too much protein, right? Actually, there is a potential for great harm eating a high-protein meat diet that can result in kidney disease, osteoporosis, cardiovascular disease, and cancers.

12) Q. If I become a vegan or raw vegan how will I get enough vitamin B12 in my diet? Doesn't B12 come from meat?

A. Most does come from meat because of the soil in the grasses the animals eat, but there is also vitamin B12 in many vegetables. You can also take an organic whole supplement. I personally use a B12 spray that I spray on my tongue every day. Back in the caveman days when people foraged for their food, they would eat some of the dirt along with their food, and as a result obtained some B12 that way. Also remember that the soil many years ago was so much better and pure than it is nowadays, so the plants were more B12 plentiful. You can also get B12 from wheatgrass therapy after a colonic when you cleanse. Adding Vitamineral Green in your green drinks or smoothies is another way to obtain B12.

13) Q. If I go off dairy how will I get enough calcium?

A. This is another huge myth out there. Your entire body chemistry changes according to the type of foods you eat. Americans' bodies have become very acidic, hence causing a variety of diseases, from cancer to tooth decay. Ideally, you want to have a PH level of 7.9 or higher. The PH scale runs from one to fourteen. For example, a soda has a PH balance of 2 which makes it extremely high in acid. Tap water has around 8.4 which is alkaline. The major acid-forming foods in our diets today include animal protein, dairy, sugar, salt, caffeine, and alcohol. Dairy products and processed foods also have the largest amounts of sodium in the American diet today. It is shown that populations that consume the highest amounts of calcium have the highest rates of osteoporosis. As explained by John A. McDougall, MD in his book *Healing Cancer from the Inside Out*, a "calcium deficiency disease" due to a low calcium intake from natural diets simply does not exist. In other words, the cause of osteoporosis is not necessarily a lack of calcium in the diet—regardless of advertising from the dairy industry. Through lobbying efforts, the dairy industry has set US standards for calcium consumption very high. The calcium scare that has been going on in this country is one of the biggest nutritional scams ever conceived. Some good organic sources of calcium:

- green drinks
- green salads
- sprouted almond milk
- sprouted wheat cereal
- raisins

- sesame seeds
- cabbage
- cucumber
- broccoli
- arugula
- bok choy
- watercress
- spinach

14) Q. Can I still drink soda or diet soda?

A. Not if you want to lose weight and get healthy. Tons of sugar, artificial sweeteners, and chemicals are added to these drinks. Drinking regular or diet soda can pack on the pounds, rot your teeth, give you headaches, and can make you sick.

Some of the most popular artificial sweeteners on the market today are:

- Splenda (sucralose)
- Aspartame
- Saccharine
- Acesulfame Potassium (acesulfame K)

These artificial sweeteners are used in abundance in almost every "diet" drink, "light" yogurts, puddings, and ice creams, most "low-carb" products, and almost all "reduced-sugar" products. Even most protein powders are loaded with artificial sweeteners (just look on the ingredients and you'll usually see one of them).

Splenda is probably one of the worst offenders of claiming-to-be-healthy artificial sweeteners, as they say that it's made from real sugar. Don't be fooled! It's still an artificial substance. What they don't tell you is that Splenda is actually a chemically modified substance where chlorine is added to the chemical structure, making it more similar to a chlorinated pesticide than something we should be eating or drinking.

The fact is, artificial sweeteners vs. sugar or corn syrup is really just a battle between two evils. Which evil is worse?

I'm sure you already know the problems with sugar or high-fructose corn syrup sweetened products. The excess empty calories, blood sugar spike, and resulting insulin surge this creates in your body not only promotes fat gain, but also stimulates your appetite further, making things even worse.

On the other hand, artificial sweeteners save you calories, but there's growing evidence that they can increase your appetite for sweets and other carbohydrates causing you to eat more later in the day anyway.

Three by-products of aspartame are methanol, formaldehyde, and formate, similar to what can be found in fruit juices. According to Michael B. Schachter MD, the methanol in juices is chemically bound so it cannot be absorbed into the body whereas in aspartame it is in a free state where it can be absorbed.

15) Q. Can I still drink alcohol?

A. As far as drinking alcohol goes, let's face it, after a couple of drinks you always want all the things you can't have. So, try only to drink organic alcohol in moderation (organic wine can be purchased at most liquor stores). If you are invited to dinner or have guests, bring a bottle with you, and share it with the group. Alcohol is also very acidic, so everything in moderation. Think about what you mix your alcohol with. Are you using soda or diet soda? There are a lot of unwanted calories and sugar in just those alone. You could also choose to have spring water with a slice of lemon or lime, or some fruit juice.

Did you know that alcohol when consumed in the body turns to a substance that is akin to embalming fluid? Acetaldehyde is the first byproduct of the body's breakdown of alcohol, and is approximately thirty times more toxic than alcohol. Used in the manufacture of adhesives and plastics, it is a close chemical cousin of formaldehyde (which is one widely-used embalming fluid). Pretty horrible, don't you think?

NINE STEPS FOR LOSING WEIGHT AND FEELING BETTER

1) Refrain from buying processed, inorganic foods out of boxes or cans.

This is not as difficult as you would think—it's the most difficult in the beginning. Obesity in the US is largely due to processed foods and the preservatives and hormones put into them, so taking these out of your diet will be a tremendous benefit. It is kind of like going back to the way our grandparents lived. They grew their own food or got it from farmers (without pesticides in the soil, or hormones given to their cows). They made things from scratch. This does make shopping easier because it just about eliminates 75 percent of the grocery isles.

2) Refrain from buying "diet" or "low-fat" foods.

Diet foods and low-fat foods only make you fat! When food manufacturers moved to marketing foods as "fat free," they added more sugar and simple (refined) carbohydrates in many products to replace the fat. So instead of eating fat, you are quickly creating fat inside your body from the added sugar. And you get cravings from the sugar, so you eat more product, etc. What a concept for the food industry, huh?

3) Refrain from eating foods with added sugar.

There is so much sugar in everything we eat these days, so preparing meals by using alternative (not artificial) sweeteners can help. Try substituting these natural organic sweeteners in place of sugar:

- raw blue agave

- stevia yacon syrup (a bit like molasses)

- organic maple syrup

- coconut crystals

- lucuma (from an exotic Peruvian fruit)

- organic raw honey

- organic unsweetened raw cocoa powder

4) Switch from table salt to organic sea salt.

This can actually make a big difference in so many ways. There are vast differences between "table salt" and organic sea salt. First, let's start with the differences. With organic sea salt:

- There is will be no feeling of bloating or water retention, and it enhances the flavors of food in a superior way to the table salt. Do a test yourself. Side by side, have your table salt and the organic sea salt. Taste one and then the other and you, too, will discover what truly exceptional salt can taste like.

- It is a whole food, as it is in nature, and contains a variety of balanced nutrients. It is loaded with mineral-rich trace elements that are essential to good health. This is important because these trace minerals satisfy your body's cravings and reduce over-eating.

- It is free of chemicals and bleach, and contains no pouring agents that deplete its nutrients. It is hand-harvested and wand solar dried, so you never get any chemicals or bleach in this salt.

- It is lower in sodium than table salt yet higher in salt flavor so you can use less. You can use more without any health worries or without losing flavor. Gourmet chefs use this salt.

- It is tested by independent laboratories so you can be sure you are getting exactly what is on the label . . . clean and pure salt.

Table salt, on the other hand, it is everything that organic sea salt is not:

- It is stripped of its precious minerals and trace elements at the processing plant.

- You have to use more of it to get the flavor you are looking for, so you eat too much of this broken-down, bleached-out, chemically-cleaned product, with very little vitamins or minerals, so-called salt.

- Salt processors and advertisers have convinced the public that we should be more concerned with the white bleached look of the product and lower costs rather than in its actual nutritional value to our bodies.

So, throw your table salt away and get some organic sea salt and enjoy salt like you never have before, without the worry of weight retention, cravings, and over-eating that regular table salt can cause.

5) Buy organic fruits, vegetables, and whole grains, and raw nuts and seeds.

They [organic and raw foods] have much more nutritional value and do not have additives or chemicals. There is a huge difference in the nutritional value you get from regular, over-the-counter fruits and veggies as opposed to organic fruits and veggies. Remember that grains should always be whole grains, not wheat mixes. It should always have the word "whole" in front of it.

When you buy organic fruits and veggies in the store, ask how the supermarket marks their organic foods. This is how it is done around my area in Massachusetts: On the stickers they put on the fruit and veggies, there will have a code in front of the PLU code (produce look up). For example:

- 4011=conventionally grown

- 84011=genetically engineered (doesn't that sound yummy?)

- 94011=organically grown

Here is some other helpful information on what "organic" really means in stores:

- 100 percent organic: must contain only organically produced ingredients.

- Organic: Defined by the USDA as containing 95 percent organic ingredients.

- Made with Organic: Must contain at least 70 percent organic ingredients. These foods cannot bear the USDA organic seal.

- Some Organic Ingredients: Products with less than 70 percent organic ingredients are only allowed to list the organic items in the ingredient panel on the side of the package. These also cannot display the USDA organic seal.

Don't confuse the label "organic" with the label "natural." They are not the same. Natural generally means that no artificial ingredients were added in processing and has nothing to do with how the product was raised or grown. Organic means that the land used to grow the food must have gone through a three-year transition period (although I have seen some places that require up to seven years) to make sure the crops are free of synthetic pesticides and synthetic fertilizers. There are also no genetically modified organisms (GMO) contained in anything labeled organic.

6) Drink filtered or distilled water rather than water from the tap.

Try not to buy the plastic container water bottles or drink water straight from the tap. The plastic in bottled water is full of PCBs (toxins), and when it breaks down, especially when they are heated up over and over again, these toxins get into the water. Ever drive by supermarkets or stores early in the morning on a hot summer day and see cases of water bottles just sitting outside in the hot sun? The plastic, especially since they started making thinner and thinner plastic bottles, is very toxic to our bodies. I have seen some water bottles that still have the thick plastic containers, but I wouldn't use them over and over again. Get yourself a glass or stainless-steel water bottle.

You can purchase a water filter that hooks up to your sink, or you can make your own. I distill my own water. You can buy a large distiller, or a small countertop distiller, which I have. I show these on my web site as well. There are filters that you change every few months. Distilled water is easy to make. When done I fill up about four large canning jars with the water. This is a lot cheaper than bottled water, and you know what you are getting.

7) Try to eliminate or cut back on meat in your diet.

If you do continue to eat meat, buy organic free-range meat and try to only consume meat one to three times weekly. All types of meat take a long time to digest and create a lot of sugar in our bodies, which is very acidic and causes so many diseases and problems in our bodies.

Check out the chart I have included on page 57 on acidic and alkaline foods. The primary acidic component of the Western diet is animal products, which are high in protein. The vast amount of plant food, however are alkaline. Even lemon juice, which you would think is acidic, is alkaline once it is in the blood stream.

A good alkaline/acid ratio for our bodies is about 80/20. But, because our diets are heavy in animal products and refined foods, it is about 20/80—totally backward.

8) Exercise at least three times weekly.

Exercise for at least forty-five minutes each time so you get a good cardiovascular work out. It is very important to keep everything working smoothly. If you want to keep healthy, you have to exercise. Start by walking for forty-five minutes to an hour three to four times a week. Then graduate to some large hills.

You can even work out at home; just keep moving! If you have time (and need some motivation), consider taking some classes at the gym (spin classes, weights, or Pilates classes, to name a few). Find a friend to walk or work out with for extra motivation.

9) Find people with similar interest in their health.

Get to know other people who eat like you. It is a great support to have others interested in the same lifestyle way of eating. Find a good food coach. I can help you with that. You can also go online and Google your eating style. There are some great online support networks to ease your transition into a healthier way of life.

TWELVE TIPS FOR LASTING RESULTS: LOSE WEIGHT FOR THE LAST TIME!

1) Do not look at this as a diet; it is a lifestyle change.

Most diets are set up to fail because they always have an end point. For example, there are those diets that say you will lose ten pounds in two weeks. So what happens after the two weeks? You go back to eating the way you did, only to gain all the weight back quickly, and often more of it than you had before. This is the unique thing about my way of eating. It is not a diet. It is a lifestyle choice, and doesn't end. That is why it works. You will see soon see that it was the best choice you ever made for yourself for getting healthy. Losing weight is just an added bonus!

When people start remarking about your weight loss and how great you look (and they will), they will ask you what diet you went on. This will happen a lot. Your reply should be that you are not on a diet but decided to make a change in the way you eat for good. The questions and looks will go away after they realize that you aren't just on a diet, but did in fact change your life style in the way you eat. Your friends and family will see you getting slimmer and fitter, and they will soon be asking you how they can do what you are doing.

2) Eat three to six times a day.

Eating infrequently only slows down your metabolism. Eating smaller meals more often revs up your metabolism and doesn't work your digestive system as hard because you are not eating a ton of food at once. It is important to eat three meals a day and two or three snacks in between them, especially if you are working out. This is a hard concept to grasp because most people think they have to eat celery and carrots and very few calories. This is a huge myth. When you start eating this way you will be thinking, *How can I possibly lose weight eating all the time?* But you do!

3) Do a cleanse twice a year.

This is not the kind that comes out of a box or can, but real food and lots of it. During the cleanse, most of the meals will be liquid meals. The other meals will be soups and salads. When you first start, it is best to do a seven to ten day cleanse. This helps you lose most of the cravings you have for sugar and caffeine. There are centers out there that will actually prepare all of the meals for you for the entire cleanse if you are too busy to do this yourself. There is a separate section for the cleanse in this book. [Note: You can also email me from my website, HealthyEating-HealthyBody.com, and I can try to put you in touch with someone who can help.].

4) Have a series of colonic hydrotherapy cleanses.

I personally recommend colonic hydrotherapy treatments when you cleanse. Finding a good colonic hydrotherapy person is the same as finding a good doctor—you get bad ones and good ones. Once you have done this cleanse, it is good to try to do a colonic once a month or at least a few times a year to keep your body in check. There is also a separate section explaining colonic cleanses as well.

5) Try to drink eight glasses of pure water daily.

This is very important for your body and health. Not only does your body thrive on water, but your brain also requires a lot of water to function every day. It also helps in the elimination process, keeping things flowing as they should, and flushing the toxins from your body. Tap water has added chlorine and fluoride; although chlorine is necessary to clean the water, the chlorine then needs to come back out of the water before drinking, which is not done through the taps. Chlorine is a toxin that should not be ingested. Fluoride is also a toxin that should not be ingested into the body, but is in many town water systems and tooth pastes. This is why a water filter should be added in your home. If you have a well, make sure that it is tested once or twice a year for bacteria. If it is found to have bacteria, then your well should also have a water filtration system added.

6) Use a weekly food chart.

A food chart will keep you on track, especially in the beginning, and make sure that you are getting enough food everyday. To keep the chart, fill out all of your meals for the whole week so you never have to think about what you are going to eat. Of course you can make changes at any time. I use this everyday and find it invaluable. For more information on how to get my food charts, you can go to my website. Every page has a week on it where you can fill in your meals and on the opposite side a powerful healthy affirmation for you. The book will hold a year's worth of weekly charts.

7) Don't eat and drink at the same time.

Allow yourself some time between eating and drinking. It is healthier for your digestive system to not mix the two. Just give about a half hour between drinking water and eating food. Everything we put in our bodies takes a certain period of time to digest, even water. The digestive tract works better by introducing certain foods in the right sequence and at different times. You can see my chart on food combining in this book on page 103.

8) To maintain focus, spend a few minutes daily on meditation or yoga.

This will help not only your digestion but will

help in a feeling of well being. Most of us live very stressful lives, and it is full of long hours. It is important for you to take time for yourself and unwind from your stressors. Do some deep breathing and stretching to bring your body back to a calm state; this allows you to continue on with the day and feel rejuvenated.

9) Be creative with meal planning.

This way, you and your family will not become bored eating the same foods all of the time. A great way to come up with new meal choices is to research your style of eating on the Internet. I have come upon a lot of great websites with wonderful new ideas. Again, using my food chart helps make the weekly food planning much easier.

10) Plan ahead when visiting others for dinner.

If you are very close, let them know ahead of time what you do not eat. You can offer to bring a large salad or healthy dessert. If you feel uncomfortable with this, just pick some of the foods that you can eat that are being offered and eat more vegetables and salad. If you are a meat eater, try to eat less of those and more veggies, some grains, and not too much dessert. I don't make a big deal about eating things you normally wouldn't when visiting friends or eating out; it's okay to go back to your eating lifestyle when you get home. Just do the best you can.

11) If you are having cravings, try to figure out why.

Maybe you missed a meal or snack? Maybe you did not drink enough water throughout the day? To alleviate a craving or urge to eat when you know you are not really hungry, drink a glass of water first and if you are still hungry, have half an apple or a handful of grapes. You can also put some almond butter on slices of apples, which is pretty filling. You should look to make sure you had enough calories during the day, especially if you are exercising more. Maybe you are not eating enough food. Listen to your body. You may need to do a cleanse if you have not done one in the past six months. If you ate some food you don't normally eat, it can trigger cravings again. They go away. Try going to sleep early or a light exercise to take your mind off food.

12) Exercise three to five times weekly.

Get out and walk, jog, bike, or go to the gym and do aerobics. Regular exercise actually keeps you from overeating. It keeps you from mistaking boredom for hunger! It also improves your wellbeing and puts you in a good mood.

FOUR THINGS IN YOUR REFRIGERATOR THAT COULD MAKE YOUR FAMILY SICK!

1) Diet soft drinks

Most diet sodas contain aspartame, which is also marketed as NutraSweet, Equal, or Amino Sweet. It is actually a neurotoxin and has been linked to brain cancer, grand mal seizures, and several other central nervous system disorders. This is a drug and it interacts with other drugs and changes the brain chemistry causing multiple types of chronic illnesses, including cancer. Plus, no one knows how long it takes to get this out of your system. The FDA has always known it was a carcinogen. Dr. Adrain Gross (FDA toxicologist) told Congress that without a doubt, Aspartame triggers brain tumors and brain cancers. Aspartame is made of three components. The first is phenylalanine, which is linked to Parkinson's disease. (Michael J. Fox was a former Diet Pepsi spokesman and suffers from this debilitating disease.) This substance cannot be metabolized, and this inability to metabolize can lead to mental retardation in children. The second substance is aspartic acid. The third substance is methanol, which is wood alcohol. Methanol is widely distributed throughout the body including the brain, muscle, fat, and nervous tissue. Methanol is toxic and can cause headaches, dizziness, nausea, ear buzzing, weakness, vertigo, chills, memory lapses, numbness, shooting pains, insomnia, depression, heart problems, pancreatic inflammation and so many other things

2) Regular milk and dairy products

Dairy products are one of the biggest reasons for allergies. Unless they are organic free range they are also full of chemicals, hormones, and preservatives, and are very acidic for our bodies. A great alternative is almond milk; you can buy it in stores or make your own.

3) Soy products

Unless they are organic soybeans these can create havoc in men and women's bodies. Many soy products are genetically modified. It is also known to influence hormones.

4) Nonorganic vegetables and fruit

If fruits and vegetables are not organic, they are sprayed with chemicals, and could be genetically modified as well; not to mention, these fruits and vegetables are devoid of many essential vitamin and minerals.

So, watch what you eat. It is a jungle out here.

FOOD CHART

HealthyEatingHealthyBody@gmail.com

ACIDIC:	ALKALINE:
A few fruits & vegetables	Almost all fruits & vegetables
All animal foods	Raw nuts
Whole & refined grains	Sprouted grains
Sugar	Herbs & spices, condiments, spicy foods
Fried food, salt	
Sodas, coffee, tea, alcohol	
Drugs, medications, tobacco	

Historical Percent of Calories:	Current Percent of Calories:
Animal foods = 5 %	Animal foods = 42 %
Refined foods = 0 %	Refined foods = 51 %
Whole plant foods = 95 %	Whole plant foods = 7 %

Reference: Anderson, Mike. *Healing Cancer from Inside Out*. 64.

Throughout our history, humans ate a diet of primarily whole, natural, alkaline plant foods. Today, whole plant foods constitute only 7 percent of our diet; 42 percent of our calories come from acidic animal foods and a whopping 51 percent of calories come from acidic refined foods.

"Is it any wonder that not only cancer, but other degenerative diseases are overtaking our bodies? In fact, it's been estimated that a whopping 70 to 85 percent of all hospital patients suffer from illnesses associated with diet-induced diseases," says Caldwell B. Esselstyn, MD.

THE DOS AND DON'TS
OF DAIRY

There is actually a good amount of research, in several populations, that shows that full-fat dairy consumption is associated with lower BMI, lower waist circumference, and lower risk of cardiovascular disease (especially stroke). Low-fat or fat-free dairy is actually often associated with increased BMI and waist circumference. Dr. Ronald Krauss, one the world's leading lipid researchers, directly shows, in the online article "What They NEVER Want You to Find Out about Real Butter," that while saturated fat from dairy does raise LDL (low-density lipoprotein, associated with cholesterol levels), it is an increase in large, fluffy, and benign LDL—not the small, dense, and atherogenic LDL. This actually decreases your risk of cardiovascular disease!

There is a clear difference between butter and dairy from cows that are fed grain and corn, milked nearly year-round, given growth hormones and antibiotics, and live in their own waste compared to cows on small farms that eat grass, get exercise, fresh air and sunshine, and are only milked based on their seasonal reproductive cycle. The quality of life, and therefore quality of milk and dairy products, is vastly different. Butter from grass-fed cows is shown to contain a lot of powerful vitamins and healthful fatty acids. These vitamins are fat-soluble, and they are bonded to the fatty acids in the dairy, and are therefore nearly non-existent in fat-free dairy. The fat is where vitamins A, D, E and K2 are, as well as a variety of other good fatty acids.

CLA (conjugated linoleic acid) is present in human body fat in proportion to dietary intake, and has been shown to be a powerful ally in the fight against cancer. Meat and dairy from grass-fed animals provide the richest source of CLA on the planet, containing three-to five-times more CLA than feedlot-raised animals. CLA has been found to greatly reduce tumor growth in animals, and possibly in humans as well.

Jo Robinson, in her book *Why Grassfed is Best! The Surprising Benefits of Grassfed Meat, Eggs, and Dairy Products*, references a Finnish study where women who had the highest levels of CLA in their diet had a 60-percent lower risk of breast cancer than those with the lowest levels. Simply switching from conventionally-raised grain-fed meat and dairy to pasture-raised grass-fed versions would have placed all the women in the lowest risk category. A good grass-fed butter will contain about 110 milligrams of CLA per tablespoon.

Several studies have found that a higher vitamin K2 (mostly from vitamin K2-MK4) intake is associated with a lower risk of heart attack, ischemic stroke, cancer incidence, cancer mortality and overall mortality. Recently, a Dutch group led by Dr. Yvonne T. van der Schouw published a paper "A High Menaquinone Intake Reduces the Incidence of Coronary Heart Disease," which examined the connection between vitamin K intake and heart attacks. It stated that men with the highest vitamin K2 consumption had a 51-percent lower risk of heart attack mortality and a 26-percent lower risk of all cause mortality compared to men consuming the lowest amount. Vitamin K2-MK4 is only found in animal products and the best known sources are grass-fed butter and fatty goose liver.

One of the ways vitamin K2 improves cardiovascular health is its ability to decrease arterial calcification by 30 to 40 percent. And, this only speaks to vitamin K2's effects of cardiovascular health; it is also crucially important for proper fetal development and bone health, to name a few additional benefits.

Dairy was the hardest thing for me to give up because I love cheese! But, it is the biggest culprit for so many problems in our lives, especially food allergies. It is easy if you have allergies to find out if it is from dairy. Take two weeks and eat no dairy products at all. That means no cow's milk, butter, cheese, or eggs. You should see a lot of them disappear probably before the two weeks is up. This is also a good test to do with your children.

Dairy also creates a lot of mucus and candida in the body. Dr. T. Colin Campbell did quite a bit of research on cancer and what causes cancer, and his research is found in *Healing Cancer from Inside Out* by Mike Anderson and *Cancer: Step Outside the Box* by Ty Bollinger. In his studies, he found that casein, which is the primary protein in all dairy products, was the most aggressive cancer promoters of all. Pretty scary ha? You do not have to have cancer to read these books, but by educating yourself and your family about this research on many of these health subjects, you may be able to prevent yourself from getting sick. These books touch on so many health issues and how to deal with them naturally.

WHAT ARE ENZYMES, AND WHY ARE THEY IMPORTANT?

It is important to know the value of the enzymes in foods and their relation to human nutrition. The truth is, we are alive only because thousands of enzymes make it possible! Enzymes are metabolism. They work twenty-four hours a day to maintain and balance our bodies. Without enzymes, we would be lifeless. All plant and animal life is full of enzyme activity. We are given a limited supply of bodily (metabolic) energy enzymes at birth, and that supply needs to last a lifetime. The faster you use up the supply, the shorter your life. Enzymes break down excess fat to be eliminated in weight loss.

It is also important to know that heat destroys all of the enzymes found in food. Of all the species on Earth, humans and our pets attempt to live without food enzymes. Food enzymes are only found in uncooked foods. Metabolic enzymes run our bodies; digestive enzymes digest our foods; and food enzymes from raw food start the digestion process. Good health depends on all the enzymes working together to ensure we get enough of them. With the lack of a lot of raw foods which have food enzymes, we have shortages and start to develop a numbers of chronic illnesses such as skin problems, allergies, obesity, certain cancers, and heart disease. Unless we continually replenish our enzymes with raw foods, our supply runs out and our health goes downhill.

You now can see the important role that enzymes play in our lives, so start adding more raw organic foods to your diet and help your body stay healthy.

THE HEALING POWER OF HEALTHY EATING

I truly believe that, given the chance, our bodies can heal themselves through proper nutrition. I am not a licensed physician or doctor but I have experienced in my own life the healing power of whole foods, and it has lead me to passionately share my experience with others.

Simplistically saying, if you cleanse your body from the inside before you start a change in the way you eat, and then include whole foods in your diet, you will be on your way to a much healthier life. By adding wheat grass, sprouts, greens, fresh fermented foods, fresh green juices, and whole grains to your diet, I believe you will improve your life, your energy level, and will be that much closer to obtaining better health and an extended life.

The US government completed two huge studies linking poor food choices with the major killers in our society: heart disease and cancer—which claim over a million American lives a year. One of these studies is called the "China Study."

Two major studies were done by the government on the effects of the American diet on health. The first study was done in 1977 and was called "Dietary Goals for the US." The second study was done in 1982 and was called "Diet Nutrition and Cancer."

These reports say the Americans eat too much sugary, salty, high-protein, and high-fat foods and not enough fresh vegetables, fruits, and whole grains. The second report goes on to also single out meat, dairy, poultry, and other cholesterol-rich foods as contributors to the increased incidence of cancer, while stating that fresh vegetables, sprouts, and greens helped to prevent cancer and other degenerative diseases. Remember this was done by our government and was well documented; it should be plastered everywhere, but it is not.

Over the last hundred years or so, Americans have gotten away from the good nourishing foods such as fresh veggies, sprouts, greens, fruits, and whole grains, which had no pesticides or chemicals in earlier decades and centuries. Instead, the American diet has continually declined and become heavily processed; chemicals are now added to the soil, and hormones are added to dairy products; grains have been stripped of their fiber and many other nutrients, and synthetic ingredients have been added back in as "fortified" for us. Really? Over 40 percent of calories in the American diet are now from saturated animal fat. This high-fat, high-sugar diet is too rich for our bodies, causing a multitude of health problems.

By cooking or processing our food, the vital nutrients are destroyed; 100 percent of their enzymes are flushed out, and vitamins, minerals, and proteins are damaged, leaving some foods with little or no nutritional value except in calories. By eating vegetables and fruits in their raw and uncooked state, they are full of nutrients, enzymes, vitamins, minerals, and proteins. By cooking them, you are virtually putting empty calories in your body devoid of all the benefits. So do you have to become RAW? No, this is not for everyone, but you can incorporate some of these raw foods into your meals and benefit dramatically.

One of my favorite quotes is from Hippocrates where he says, "Let your food be your medicine, and medicine be our food." He was a very wise man! There have been hundreds of drugless healers for thousands of years from ancient Greece to Eastern medicine throughout Asia dating back at least 5,000 years B.C.E. Chemotherapy, pharmaceuticals, and surgeries are modern-day replacement for natural treatments of years ago. We need to go back to our roots of many years ago and start treating our bodies with good clean, nutritional food from the beginning of our lives, rather than prescription drugs, which often create more uncomfortable side effects and problems than they relieve. Drugs and modern medicines will make you feel better but they don't heal the problems—just the symptoms. They just put a Band-Aid on them. A lot of your ailments can go away just by eating right and cleansing your insides from old waste. Don't you think it is funny when you see a new drug commercial and more than half of it is dedicated to warnings and side effects?

Healing yourself through food is slower than taking a pill to make you feel better, but there aren't any side effects and you actually get better (rather than simply feeling better). Our society is so used to getting quick results regardless of the cost to our bodies, but many people are beginning to think the doctors from centuries ago had it right—treat the body by what you put in it. We tend to believe everything our doctors tell us, but they are simply teaching what they have been taught. Doctors are not really required to get a nutritional license, so, some don't understand the full impact of proper nutrition. Can it really be this simple? Eating right? Yes, it can. We are all just so used to being told what is right for our bodies from the food pyramid put out by the government, which is now considered to be completely wrong. We take everything at face value and believe our doctors always know best. The truth is that we all need to take responsibility for our own health if we want to stay out of the hospital, off drugs and prescriptions, and keep our organs healthy.

DIFFERENCES BETWEEN EATING STYLES
The Meat Eater
The Vegetarian
The Vegan and Raw Vegan

The Meat Eater

I remember when I used to eat meat. My favorite meals were roast beef, chicken, hamburgers, and veal (until I found out that it was a baby calf). I used to love the taste of meat and the smells. I still like the smell of a good steak grilling on the BBQ, or chicken broiling in the oven. There are lots of meats associated with the way we eat in our society, such as baseball tagged with the hotdog; the Fourth of July with hamburgers, hot dogs, chili, and sausages; and Thanksgiving with turkey or ham. The list goes on and on.

It seems there is a fast food restaurant around every corner these days. Life in the United States makes it very easy for us to just grab fast food. It is no wonder there are so many unhealthy people in our society today, but there are some small changes you can do to help you get a healthier while still enjoying being a meat eater. You just need to make some adjustments to help you along.

One easy change you can make is to switch to free-range organic meat. A lot of people don't realize the difference of how cows and chickens live and get fed on an organic, free-range farm, as opposed to how they live and get fed on a farm that is not free range.

As explored in the movie *Food Inc.*, dairy cows are usually in one place all day on a non-free-range farm. Some of them can no longer even walk. The cows are fed a lot of corn products (which are usually genetically modified) to fatten them up; this is not their natural food source. Some of them even have openings in their throats for the farmers to clean out the byproducts of the corn products because they cannot digest this unnatural food. Dairy cows are also fed hormones to increase production of milk and antibiotics to keep them from getting sick, which are then passed onto humans when we consume their products. There are studies that show that children are going through adolescence much earlier, and it is suspected that the cause is the hormones in our dairy and meat.

Organic free-range dairy cows do not have hormones or antibiotics in their milk, which in turn makes the milk much healthier and safer to consume. This makes all dairy products healthier from these cows. These cows are put out in organic pastures where they eat what Mother Nature intended—grass!

Most chickens that are not raised organic and free-range, be it for egg or for meat, never see the light of day and usually packed in so tightly that their environment is totally filthy, causing filth and disease. They are also fed corn and other byproducts, which are unnatural food sources for them. Free-range organic chickens, on the other hand, run outside eating their natural food sources without pesticides and chemicals. As a result of this, these chickens' eggs are also much healthier for you. This is also a much more humane way of treating our animals.

Everyone should be aware of what dietary choices they are making. In this case, it is important that meat eaters be aware of the differences between meat from organic free-range sources and everyday supermarket meat. Cows are made to eat grass, and chickens are meant to eat grass and bugs out in the open fresh air. That is all they need. So purchasing organic free-range meat and dairy is not only healthier, it is also an ethical thing to do.

Some ideas for becoming a healthier meat eater:

- Consider decreasing the amount of meat you eat in a week. This will also help to offset the price difference in eating organic meat and dairy.

- You can also start cutting down on your portion size of your meat. Most Westerners eat way too much meat and protein; the protein you get from meat products (which is acidic) is a lot harder on the body to digest, as opposed to the protein you get from vegetables (which is alkaline based). It is important to know this because, when your body is working overtime trying to digest meat products, it is very hard on the body and it takes away from being able to keep up with digesting your food properly. Eating less meat and dairy gives your body a break. You will probably also find that you have a lot less indigestion when eating less meat, thus cutting back on the over-the-counter antacids.

- Start adding more organic vegetables to your meals. This will fill you up while giving you added fiber, vitamins, and nutrients and fewer fat and calories.

- Try to drink a lot more pure water throughout the day. Shoot for at least eight glasses a day. This will keep you full and hydrated as well. Often times, people mistake being hungry from actually just being thirsty. Try not to drink water or other liquids within thirty minutes before or after eating, as this challenges the digestion. Drinking enough water can cut cravings for meat.

- Switch your table salt for organic sea salt. Most people who eat meat really load on the salt, so using organic sea salt is not only better for you, but it is stronger (so you don't need as much) and tastes a lot better. Regular salt has been processed chemically and bleached, and it really has very little nutritional value left.

- Eat three meals daily and one to three snacks. When you are eating every three hours, you are avoiding hunger, your metabolism is always working, and your body won't get overloaded by large meals. This way you will not be tempted to overeat on your meat portions.

- Try to do a seven-to ten-day cleanse a couple of times a year to flush out excess waste and toxins from your body

- Men and Women should do a series of colonic cleanses a few times a year to clean out old undigested food. This is especially important for meat and dairy eaters. Because meat and dairy are harder to digest and are very acidic, a lot of the meat products are never fully released from your body, which in turn creates a large amount of undigested waste buildup in your body over the years. This is what causes a lot of sickness and disease. By removing this waste with a series of these colonics, you are going to feel incredibly better and your body will be able to start repairing and healing itself. See page 97 for more information on colonics.

The Vegetarian

I became a vegetarian when I was twenty-one years old. It was also back in the hippie days, and being a vegetarian was very popular at the time. It took a bit of adjustment going off red meat, but I did. Though I still occasionally ate a limited amount of chicken and fish, but identified myself with as a lacto-ovo vegetarian eating style (which meant I still occasionally consumed dairy products and eggs). I remember eating a lot of brown rice, which I cooked from scratch, a lot more vegetables, I stopped drinking milk, but I did eat cheese. I also stopped eating white bread and a lot of unhealthy desserts. I ate beans to replace my protein loss.

Being hungry all of the time is one thing I remember about first becoming a vegetarian. I thought I was going to get fat eating so much food, but I never did. Eating a lot of meals a day was not something I had ever done before. So when I had fried rice and vegetables for lunch, I was hungry three hours later. I adjusted after a couple of weeks and felt safe eating whenever I was hungry.

I lost weight, which was a big surprise to me considering how much I was eating. My health also improved quite a bit. Getting sick was very infrequent and I had a lot of energy. Eating this lifestyle fit right in with where I was at the time. I do remember that every time I tried to give blood I was turned down for anemia, indicating that I was not getting enough iron in my blood. But, I stayed as a vegetarian until I was fifty-four years old. That is hard to see on paper as I am writing this. I am now sixty, but I really feel like I am in my twenties.

Some ideas for becoming a healthier vegetarian:

- Try to incorporate more raw foods into your diet. If I had done this when I was a vegetarian, I most likely would not have been anemic. By cooking all of your foods, you are actually killing the wonderful enzymes that are in raw foods naturally. You are also killing a lot of the vitamins and minerals. Raw foods are packed full of vitamins, minerals, nutrients, fiber, and enzymes. When you cook them, a lot of those disappear.

- Eat organic vegetables, fruits, and nuts. The differences between organic and nonorganic foods are huge! Organic foods come from nutritional soil which makes your food much more nutrient rich; dangerous chemicals, pesticides, and hormones do not exist in organic foods; organic foods are also not genetically altered.

- Make sure you are drinking a lot of filtered water for hydration and digestion.

- Try to buy organic coffee and teas and wine if you drink them.

- Try to eat three meals a day and one to three snacks so your digestion will be on track, and you won't feel hungry during the day.

The Vegan or Raw Vegan

Both vegan diets consist of food that is organically grown, using no dairy, fish, meat, or animal products. Raw vegans generally do not cook their food. Do they eat cooked food sometimes? Yes, but the bulk of their food is uncooked or warmed between 105—112 degrees Fahrenheit. The reason for this is that the enzymes in food are killed above this temperature, so you are not benefiting from them or a lot of other vitamins. Once I started eating raw, I noticed that things I used to eat tasted better. I love it when I take a handful of fresh, homemade sprouts. The crunch and "alive" taste is wonderful to me. Kind of like how I felt when I used to bite into a juicy hamburger, or chicken. My taste buds are very much in tune with nature and what it has to offer me in the raw form.

The biggest misconception people have about this way of eating is they think that raw vegans just eat salads every day. Nothing could be further from the truth. With the influx of raw vegans in the United States today, there has been a lot of creativity with meals. There are wonderful raw vegan gourmet chefs as well. Different salads, sandwiches, soups, raw chocolate, ice cream, and desserts are things I eat being a raw vegan. There is a lot of good stuff to eat out there!

I have gained a new appreciation for eating and enjoying food now that I eat raw and organic. First of all, the taste is wonderful. If you do not eat lots of raw foods, you may have to acquire a taste for it. With any change this would happen. After you start eating this way and go into a restaurant or someone cooks your veggies to death, the other food just doesn't taste good any more. You also learn to chew your food better. This isn't something I ever thought about before until I became a raw vegan. When food is in its natural state, it is full of fiber and takes a while to chew. I remember when I used to eat my food it generally was gone in five to ten minutes because I was always in a hurry. It also was easier and quicker to eat because most of it was processed or cooked. Have you ever eaten white bread, and then also had a slice of whole-grain bread? You can definitely feel and taste the difference. In whole-grain bread, there is more substance and it takes a bit longer to chew.

You also feel fuller while eating whole grains.

For breakfast some days, I will have raw granola with organic blueberries and apples, hemp seeds for protein, and almond milk. With a regular out-of-the-box cereal from the supermarket I would have scoffed it down in five minutes. Eating my raw granola takes me twenty to thirty minutes to eat. You start appreciating the food you are eating, and you will begin loving the tastes. And, you are satisfied and full afterward.

Like any way of eating, you want to make sure you are getting everything your body requires and needs. This is no different. There are different vitamins and minerals in different foods, so it is important to eat a variety of things. The list below I have incorporated into my daily lifestyle and are good things to include in yours as well.

Some ideas for becoming a healthier vegan or raw vegan:

- Make sure you drink at least eight glasses of filtered water a day to aid digestion and keep hydrated.

- Eat a variety of organic fruits and vegetables during the week. Your choices will change with the seasons as well.

- Eat a variety of organic nuts and seeds from almonds, walnuts, or brazil nuts, to sesame seeds, pumpkin seeds, etc.

- Try to eliminate caffeine and sodas. Other than smoothies and green drinks, water is my choice. If there is a special occasion, I will have a bit of organic red wine.

- Eliminate added sugar and table salt from your life. You can use organic sea salt in place of table salt, and other organic sweeteners as you need them, which I have mentioned in a separate section in this book.

- Cut soy products out of your diet. They are over processed. If I do eat a soy product it is rare, and the product will be real organic soybeans.

- Incorporate whole grains or sprouted grains into your diet.

- Drink a green smoothie every day. Directions for making these on page 113.

- Drink a fruit smoothie every day. Directions for making these on page 109.

- Do a seven-to ten-day cleanse twice a year. This is discussed more fully on page 97.

- Do a series of colonics a couple of times a year. This is discussed more fully on page 99.

INTRODUCING HEALTHY EATING
TO THE FAMILY

Here are some common fears and concerns people have about making healthy changes in the family's diet. This is totally normal and to be expected; no one really likes change in the beginning.

- Everyone likes something different.

- I don't have time to make this kind of food.

- I have picky eaters.

- It is going to cost a lot more to eat healthy.

- I will have to learn how to make these things and fit it into my already-busy schedule.

These are all good concerns, and important ones to look at. I think the first thing you need to look at is how important is your family's health? Would it be worth it for your family if you took a little extra time preparing things from scratch if it meant that all of you would benefit greatly from that? What if, by making some healthy changes, it actually improved your family's health and they weren't sick as much, or their allergies went away? What if it allowed your family members to have longer, fuller lives? In the long run this will save you time and money, and make for a much happier family.

When I first became a raw vegan I didn't know where I would find the time to do it. But I found that this eating style is like anything else that is new . . . a new job, a new place to live, or a new baby. It is mostly difficult in the beginning because you are not used to it. I had my challenges when I first started, as it was new and different and I have a busy work schedule. But after I did it for a week or two, I found that it wasn't that hard after all.

I didn't have the challenges that a lot of families have, as my son was already in college when I made this change, but he did live with me during the summer. I didn't push him at all, but I found that he wanted to keep trying more and more of my food. By the time he went back to school, he became a vegan. Two weeks after he left for school. he called me and said that he could smell again. He had not been able to smell well for years, and giving up dairy did the trick. He is still a vegan today after three years.

When I was in my early twenties, I was raising my boyfriend's two children. When they moved in with us, I decided that we would all be vegetarians. That didn't go over well because it was done in one step, and by force. I have learned a lot since then. You can't force someone to eat a certain way, and if you want to help people change the way they eat, you introduce things slowly to them and let them decide for themselves.

You may be thinking to yourself, *How can I possibly be a raw vegan or vegan when I have three children and a spouse?* First of all, being a vegan or raw vegan is not for everyone. There may be some members of your family who want to be vegetarians, some that embrace being a vegan, and some that will never give up eating meat and dairy. Getting your family on board may have its difficulties but you don't have to turn the family into vegans or raw vegans entirely. You can just add some healthier food in addition to what they are already eating and replace some of the food that is not very healthy for them.

Try slowly adding more healthy organic foods with your current meals, and offering alternatives to sugar drinks and dairy. Make a plan for yourself and have everyone chip in and help once a week to start. Let them be part of some fun meal planning. Schedule out the changes you plan to make so that your family has time to prepare.

The first things you should do:

- Get a water filter on the counter, on your water spigot, or in the refrigerator if it dispenses water. Or you could put a water filter under the kitchen sink so it is easier for everyone to grab a fresh glass of water. Make sure you change filters every few months.

- Keep jars of cold, pure water in the refrigerator to encourage your family to drink it. Make lemonade using filtered water instead of buying the kind with sugar and additives. When you make your own, also use organic lemons and a sugar alternative, such as organic honey or organic maple syrup. This water can also make a big difference with coffee and tea!

- Make your ice cubes with filtered water as well. Unlike with tap water, distilled or filtered water has no aftertastes.

- Buy organic coffee and tea brands. These last few suggestions they will hardly notice if you make it an everyday thing.

- Start replacing diet drinks and sodas of all kinds with natural organic juices and pure sparkling waters. Sodas of any kind are absolutely the worst things you can drink

- Pack water for the kids when they go to school. Get them nice cool water containers.

- Throw away your table salt and get an organic sea salt. You don't need as much, it tastes better, and is better for you.

- Throw away the sugar and put an organic sweetener in its place. You can even have an assortment of different organic sweeteners, some powder, some granular, and some liquid, something for everyone. Put an alternative granulated sweetener in the sugar bowl and they probably won't even notice the difference. I have mentioned the alternative sweeteners in this book. You can also use these things to cook or make your meals with instead of the old stuff.

- Offer organic salads, large ones full of greens, sprouts, and anything else you can think to put in them, like walnuts, almonds, grapes, apples, avocados with all of your meals. Add some raw vegetables in the salad or as finger food. Good ones are fresh carrots (not the small ones that are peeled), raw broccoli (which a lot of kids like raw much better than cooked), some sliced raw zucchini, red and yellow peppers, etc. Start out with just a few and add more as the weeks go on. Make them colorful, and have an array of organic salad dressings. If your family is adverse to trying organic foods, start out by putting them in a glass dressing server so they do not all see that it is organic. Often times, people resist things that are different.

- Have fresh organic raw finger vegetables in the refrigerator as snacks. You can also have organic dips to enhance their flavor.

Over the next three months add some additional new foods, just a little at a time:

- Replace cow's milk with nut milk, such as almond milk. You can make your own (make sure the nuts are organic and raw, not salted or processed in any way) or purchase but milk in the supermarket. (Of course, make sure no one is allergic to almonds.) Making it is less expensive and I have the recipe on page 111. You can use but milk with anything that calls for milk in your recipes, like mashed potatoes or desserts. You really can't tell the difference.

- If you can't quite give up milk, buy organic free-range milk. It is more expensive but so much healthier for you.

- You can start out making these changes without letting anyone know. If they ask, just say you are trying a new recipe or just say you wanted to try something healthier.

- Just add a new item every few days and incorporate into the menu.

- If your family eats meat and eggs, start buying organic free-range; it will only taste better.

- Buy fish that is fresh from the oceans or rivers and not hatcheries where they are fed unnatural, processed fish food. Try to stay away from fish high in mercury. If you fry your fish, use good organic olive oil.

- When you get eggs and butter, get free-range organic. These particular things are a bit more expensive, but they are so much healthier for you.

- Start cooking whole foods instead of buying packaged foods that are processed and lifeless. Not only are whole foods healthier for you, they taste better. Try getting organic whole-grain rice and spaghetti. It is thicker, but it also isn't pasty like the regular, white, devoid-of-fiber kind you usually get.

- Instead of packaged macaroni and cheese, make your own. Make a lot and freeze it so you have extra for another night. This will save you time.

Over the first six months and beyond:

- Continue adding more raw vegetables with dinners.

- Start serving smaller servings of meat and fish. Your ultimate goal is to make it so everyone is eating more vegetables (so use some steamed and some raw, so you are getting your nutrients) and smaller amounts of starches, such as potatoes, spaghetti, and bread.

- This would also be a good time to offer a choice of whole grain bread with meals along with the traditional white. Try to get your family to try this healthier and more filling bread.

- As far as cost goes, if you started eliminating the junk food and sodas, and all of the packaged food that you buy, that would be your savings! If you cut back on the amount of meat and dairy you eat, that would be a savings as well. You can spend that money that you normally spend on food that has no nutritional value on good food for the family. When everyone is eating healthier, your family will start to also get healthier; they will be sick less often, and will not need the doctor's office, medicines, and over the counter products as often as before. That is a huge savings.

- Involve the family in preparing the food. Make it fun. A. Or give one person the whole menu. Just give a bit of guidance telling them that there needs to be some vegetables, starch, and protein.

- Start encouraging your kids and spouses to learn and watch shows about the benefits of eating healthier, and shows about what happens to your body when you eat certain foods. What diseases are caused by some of the food we eat? Go together to a farmer's market once a week and everyone pick out foods to prepare for the week. Go shopping with the kids and walk around the outside of the supermarket isles where all of the fruits and veggies are. Maybe buy some easy-read books on nutrition or certain types of eating styles.

- As your kids to Google some of their favorite celebrities and their eating styles (like vegetarian, vegan, and raw vegan).

- Get a good colorful vegan or vegetarian cookbook and have everyone pick out a few that they would like to try. You can pick each person's favorite and rotate. Get involved and get the family involved.

- To save time making my food, make two days' worth of smoothies, three days' worth of green juice, three days' worth of salad, a week's worth of sprouts, dehydrated crackers for the week, a batch of veggie burgers, and falafels. These are only some steps you can do. When I make my food, I take a day to "un-cook," so I spend around four hours making all of the food I mentioned. So there are quite a few days I am not making food at all.

- Make a huge salad every time you make one so it lasts you for days. (Just don't put the tomatoes or dressings on the greens. Keep them in separate containers so the salad lasts longer.)

- Steam your veggies if you are cooking them and add either oil, vegan butter (a natural heart-healthy spread made with a blend of expeller-pressed oils shown to raise good cholesterol while lowering bad), or organic free-range butter.

- Try replacing some packaged foods with whole food products. Look at the box and see the amount of sugar and salt they contain as well as artificial colors and things you can't pronounce.

- Buy or make organic granola. Make a huge batch and then keep it in air-tight containers. Your family will love that. You can add some almond milk and fresh or frozen organic fruits.

- Throw away the instant breakfast, including oatmeal, and pick up organic whole-grain oats. It only takes twenty minutes to cook, and it will last a couple of days for another meal. You can also buy chia seeds, which are packed full of protein! It makes a food like cream of wheat, and goes a long way—a tablespoon will make about half a cup. Just pour hot water on top until it reaches the consistency you desire. Add cinnamon and a natural sweetener if you like, and some fruit and almond milk.

- There are also organic pancake mixes made from buckwheat etc. that you mix with water that are delicious! Throw some blueberries in and top with organic maple syrup or agave.

- You can make a batch of smoothies with frozen bananas and blueberries. I have the recipe in this book. This will be a big hit with everyone in the family. And you can get creative by using different fruit, etc.

- Soups also make great dinners or lunches. You can buy organic soups or you can make your own using almond milk, or filtered water, sea salt, organic vegetables, organic free-range meat, etc.

- Introduce whole-grain sprouted bread
  and organic butter. Regardless of how you
  decide to eat, it is a good idea to eliminate
  white bread from your diet. There are a lot
  of whole-grain breads out there. There are
  also breads in the freezer section which are
  whole-grain sprouted, and much easier to
  digest. They also make sprouted English
  muffins, which are great. But in any case,
  bread is bread and too much is not good for
  the waist line. So cut back on it. You will
  find that whole-grain bread is more filling
  than the white breads or mixes. There is also
  a bread called Mana bread, which is very
  good for you. Try adding nut butters on it
  instead of sugary toppings.

- When putting the food on the plates, make
  sure the veggies take up a good portion, then
  pasta and potatoes or yams not taking up
  as much space as in the past, then a smaller
  portion than you normally eat of meat
  or fish.

- By eating organic salads and vegetables, you
  are going to be getting more protein and
  nutrients. Try adding organic spinach as
  well, as it is also high in protein. Some kids
  don't like cooked spinach, so try the raw
  spinach first. It tastes completely different,

and they may like it in their salad or smoothies (which they won't taste at all).

- I notice that a lot of people eat fruit for dessert. You should change this habit. Because fruit does not take a long time to digest, it will sit in your stomach and ferment while your high-protein and high-fiber meal, which was eaten first, takes time to digest.

- Have some healthy snacks around the house at all times. Put them in little baggies or containers so they are portion controlled and easy to grab. These can consist of nuts; trail mix; fresh fruit or dried fruit; or peanut-butter or almond-butter rolls with raisins, coconut, and seeds with some sweetener if need be. For the rolls, mix ingredients together and put in round rolls. Kids love them.

If you are getting pressured by the family about incorporating these new eating styles, try compromising. Perhaps each person gets a night to make what they like for the family. So meat (if they eat meat) one night, vegetarian another, and vegan or raw vegan for another. Ask them to be patient as you introduce more foods into their lives and ask them to give it a month to see how everyone is feeling.

WEEKLY FOOD CHART:

HealthyEatingHealthyBody@gmail.com

DATE:	BREAK:	SNACK:	LUNCH:	SNACK:	DINNER:	SNACK:
MON:						
TUES:						
WED:						
THURS:						
FRI:						
SAT:						
SUN:						

WOULD YOU LIKE TO LOSE FIVE TO TEN POUNDS IN TEN DAYS?
Well, you could just by doing a cleanse!

The Cleanse

There are a lot of cleanses out there on the market these days. Most come in a box or bottle. I do not recommend these cleanses. I recommend a cleanse that is wholesome, real food, not the stuff in the box or the "quick fixes." There are health and wellness clinics out there that will make your food for you during the cleanse or show you how, and will sometimes do the colonics for you as well. I have those on my web site as well. I also recommend pairing the colonics with the cleanse. You will see maximum results this way. During the cleanse, you will not be starving yourself, as on a lot of cleanses. You will be eating about six times a day. If this is your first cleanse I recommend doing a seven-to ten-day cleanse, and then you can do a three-to five-day cleanse once or twice a year (your regular tune-up).

Not only will you lose weight on this cleanse, you will also lose a lot of cravings for sugar and caffeine. You will probably experience headaches for the first two to three days depending on how much junk you eat. They will go away. It is just your body detoxing. The food you can expect to eat on one of these cleanses is vegan. So if you do eat meat or are a vegetarian, remember, it is only for seven to ten days and you will definitely feel better and should not be hungry at all.

The typical food you will eat on the cleanse will consist of:

- sixteen ounces of green juices (throughout the day)

- eight glasses of filtered water

- an apple or two

- raw soup, which can be warmed to under 105 degrees

- a large salad full of greens, sprouts, all kinds of veggies, avocado, and organic salad dressing

- a fruit smoothie

- a delicious probiotic drink

You will be eating something about every three to four hours even if you are not hungry. What is great about the place I have my cleanse in New-buryport, Massachusetts is that they make all of the food for you for the entire cleanse. You come in and pick up your food every two to three days, or they deliver it if you live within a reasonable distance. The food is well marked and comes in a cute, easy-to-manage hot/cold bag. It truly could not be any easier! If you decide to come to Newburyport to do these cleanses, they can refer you to a couple of places to stay that they have arranged with different inns at a discounted rate. There are quite a few people who travel from all over the United States for these cleanses. If you are interested in knowing how to get in touch with them, you can find their information on my web site at www.Healthy EatingHealthyBody.com

The Colonic

Before starting any change in diet, it is important to prepare your body first. Just as you would give your car a tune-up a few times a year, so it is with the body. If you only pour more oil in your car when it is time for an oil change, you will be pouring good oil on top of sludge, and this will lessen the life of your engine. So it is with the body. You need to get all of the old "sludge," or waste, out of your colon. Your intestines are very long and hold years of old matter in them. According to Dr. Scott Whitaker, a naturopathic doctor, Elvis had twenty-two pounds of toxic fecal matter and sludge in his colon when he passed away. John Wayne's autopsy revealed that his colon weighed eighty-two pounds; seventy-seven pounds were composed of dried fecal matter, and the remaining five pounds was living tissue.

There could be many years' worth of old waste in your colon there, and it just doesn't come out by itself. It needs to be removed. By keeping the old waste in your body, it promotes disease and sickness and weakens your organs and colon. Having a series of colonics is the best way to cleanse your body. This should be done at least once a year.

Starting a new way of eating as a life choice with proper nutrition with enzymes and vitamins from live foods is not enough to ensure good health and reversal of disease or health issues. A thorough body cleansing with colonics is just as important and necessary. During this process, you will probably remove metabolic wastes, mucus, fat, calcium, excess protein, and all kinds of heavy metals (such as aluminum, lead, mercury etc.), chemical residuals from food additives, drugs, sprays, radiation from x-rays, and pollution.

A colonic is not the same as a colonoscopy, which can be very dangerous. Colonics are also not enemas, and they require a professional with professional equipment to administer them. A colonic is usually done in a spa-like room, where water is introduced into the body for about forty-five minutes, entering and releasing during this period of time. Old waste is broken down in the intestinal walls and easily removed through this procedure. I was very hesitant and scared to this at first because I thought it would be too embarrassing or it would hurt. I was worried about noises and smells, etc. It was nothing like I thought. When you are there, there is quite music playing in the background, you are covered by a sheet, and you do not hear or smell anything at all. I have only had good experiences when I have had colonics, and I feel absolutely wonderful afterward. It is totally painless. You can find a professional on my website.

Summing Up the Cleanse and the Colonic

If you are going to change the way you eat in order to get healthy, you are not doing it fully without doing a cleanse and a colonic. Having these colonics will make you healthier and help prolong your life. If you have eaten badly over the years, junk food, processed foods, a lot of meat and dairy, there is likely a lot of toxins built up in your body. You should never make a huge eating change in your life without first doing a series of colonics paired with a seven-to ten-day organic, natural cleanse. I certainly would not. Even if you are not making any changes to your diet, you should really consider colonics. They are the best thing to do for your body and for your health. Just make sure that the company doing the colonics is reputable.

The sooner your body is cleansed of all the toxins and waste products, the sooner your body will reward you in repairing itself and giving you your health back. A lot of those aches, pains, colds, flues, allergies, etc. will just disappear. So, what are you waiting for? If you want to see the best and most beneficial results for your health and body, do the colonics and a seven-to ten-day cleanse together first, then proceed with your new healthy way of eating.

A GUIDE TO COMBINING FOODS

Poor Combinations:

- fruits and most vegetables
- proteins and most starches
- two different type of proteins together
- proteins and fats
- two different starches together
- nuts or seeds (protein) with fruit

General Rules of Proper Food Consumption:

- Do not eat after 8:00 p.m. (though there will always be exceptions).
- Do not combine dense proteins and starches.

- Do not combine acid fruits with sweet fruits.

- Eat fruits alone or blended with greens only.

- Melons are best eaten alone, not mixed with other fruits (except watermelon).

- Drink liquids alone and try to wait about half an hour before eating.

- Only have one protein and one fat per meal.

FOODS THAT COMBINE WELL

Oily Proteins:

- coconuts
- nuts
- seeds
- avocados

Starches:

- sprouted grains
- yams and potatoes
- corn
- squash
- lima beans

Low-starch Veggies and Sprouts:

- leafy greens (romaine lettuce, kale, etc.)
- cabbage
- colorful peppers
- cucumbers
- celery
- broccoli
- cauliflower
- sprouts

Cultured Foods:

- seed cheeses
- sauerkraut
- pickles and relish

HOW LONG DOES FOOD REMAIN IN THE STOMACH?

HealthyEatingHealthyBody@gmail.com

Juice:	15–30 minutes
Wheat grass:	15–30 minutes
Fruit:	30–60 minutes
Water:	10–15 minutes
Most vegetables:	1– 2hours
Nuts, seeds:	2–3 hours
Sprouts:	1 hour
Melons:	60–90 minutes
Meat and fish:	3–4 hours
Beans and grains:	1–2 hours
Parley:	15 minutes
Avocado:	1.5 Hours-2 hours
Coconut milk:	2 hours
Shell fish:	8 or more hours

Reference: "Composition and Facts about Foods," *Diet Digest*.

RECIPES FOR HEALTHY STAPLES

Fruit Smoothie

My favorite smoothie can be changed around to your taste; use different fruit, add some things, or take things out for a different flavor.

Ingredients:

- 1 ½ organic frozen bananas (peel the bananas and then freeze them in bags)
- 1 cup of organic frozen blueberries (I like Wyman's brand as they come in large bags in the freezer section of most grocery stores)
- 2 cups of coconut water (or you can use one part coconut water, one part filtered water)
- ½ tablespoon raw chocolate nibs
- 1 tablespoon cinnamon
- 1 tablespoon vita-mineral greens (optional)
- 1 tablespoon hemp seeds for protein (optional)
- 1 date role (optional)
- Handful of organic spinach (don't worry you don't taste the veggies at all)

Directions:

Blend at high speed for about two to three minutes. Pour into two sixteen-ounce jars and keep in frig until you use them. They will last two to three days and that will make about three to four smoothies.

Note: You can also make fruit smoothies using strawberries, raspberries, blueberries, vanilla, etc. Just mix them up. Kids love them!

Nut Milk

To make almond milk, hazelnut milk, or a number of other types of nut milk, you only need few things: a nut bag, a large wide-mouth thirty-two-ounce canning jar, a plastic cover with holes in the top (or a cheese cloth), pure distilled water, and some raw organic almonds or other nuts of your choice (not salted or roasted). It is very simple to do and only takes about five minutes. This recipe is for one large canning jar of almond milk. On my website, I list places you can get supplies.

Ingredients:

¼ cup raw almonds (or other raw nuts)
pure distilled or filtered water

Directions:

Take the raw almonds (or another raw nut) and soak them in about eight ounces of pure distilled or filtered water for about six hours. Then drain the nuts well a few times to get the peelings off. Put the nuts in a blender (if you soak more almonds you can put the rest in a covered jar in the refrigerator for later use). Fill the large canning jar with filtered water, minus about ¼ of a cup (so not quite all the way to the top). Pour water and nuts in blender and blend at high speed for one to two minutes. Take a wide, shallow bowl and put the empty canning jar in the middle of it. Take out your cheese cloth and place it over the mouth of the jar; pour mixture into the jar, the cheese cloth sifting out the nuts. Put any spilled-over milk from the bowl into the jar. Cover with an airtight lid, and put in the refrigerator.

Nut milk is great with cereals, coffee, tea, oatmeal, mashed potatoes, and anything you normally use regular milk with, chocolate milk, etc. It tastes great, and kids love it. You can make this milk thicker or thinner just by adding or reducing the amount of water. This is less expensive than buying milk or premade nut milk. You also don't have to worry about milk intolerance, it is less fattening and higher in protein than cow's milk, and is a lot more nutritious than cow's milk. If your family drinks a lot of milk, you can double or triple the recipe—just make sure to have enough canning jars!

Green Smoothie

This will make two large sixteen-ounce canning jars' worth of juice, which is good for two days, or one if you are cleansing.

Ingredients:

1 ½ bunch of celery

2 large cucumbers

½ of a granny smith apple

1 small piece of ginger (about one tablespoon)

1 cup of spinach

1 bunch of kale, romaine lettuce, Swiss chard, or any seasonal greens

½ cup of sprouts (optional)

1 small bunch of parsley (I like curly)

2 large carrots (optional)

1 small beet (optional)

Directions:

Put all ingredients into a juicer so the pulp comes out separate from the liquid. If you dehydrate foods, you can use the pulp in with different recipes. This will take you about twenty minutes to juice and another five to ten minutes to clean the juicer afterward. Put into two canning jars and refrigerate. You can use different greens in this recipe. I like a light-tasting juice. Change it up for your taste. Have one sixteen-ounce jar a day, or two of them if you are cleansing.

Sprouts

These are the easiest and least expensive food to grow, and they are full of nutrition, enzymes, vitamins, minerals, chlorophyll, and protein. Having your children make these would be a great project! They can be used in about everything. You can eat them as they are, or put them in salads, sandwiches, casseroles, smoothies, or just treat them as a snack. With the scare of E. coli surrounding store-bought sprouts, it is another good reason to make them yourselves. They do not require much attention either.

I sprout every four to five days and use the following sprout seeds and beans, but there are others you can choose to use:

- mung beans

- green lentils

- adzuki beans

- alfalfa seeds

- clover

- wheat berries

Directions:

Sprouts poof when they grow, so they will fill a jar. Put about one to two inches of seeds in the bottom of the jar, and fill up the jar with filtered water. Let them sit for about six hours; then, rinse them well a few times, and drain the water. Place the jar directly in the sunlight and watch the sprouts grow.

I only purchase these seeds organically from a local market or organic store. You can get them in bulk, and they can stay in the refrigerator for a good amount of time before you use them. Just don't get them wet.

It is very important to purchase your seeds or beans organically so you know they won't be tainted. When you buy sprouts in the stores, they go through a process of handling by many people, and you don't know in what environment they were grown, whether their facility was clean, the soil had pesticides and chemicals, etc. This is why it is best to grow sprouts yourself. It truly is easy, inexpensive, and fun to grow them.

In the winter, it can take four to five days to sprout the seeds. In the summer, because it is warmer, it usually takes three to four days depending on the size of the seeds. You can also mix different seeds, but just remember to put the same size seeds together when growing. As an example, I grow mung beans and lentils together because they are around the same size. If you are growing clover, they are smaller seeds, so you could them grow with alfalfa seeds which are very similar in size.

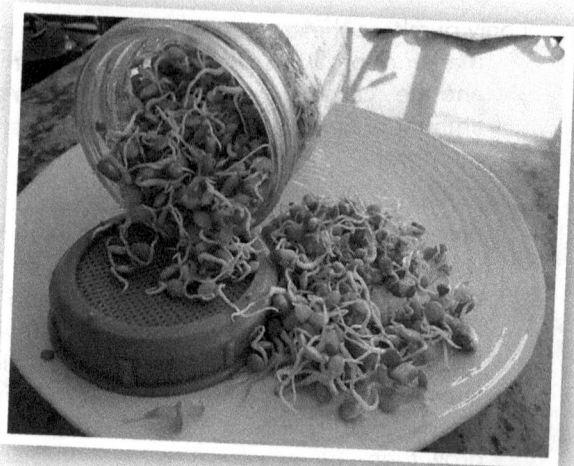

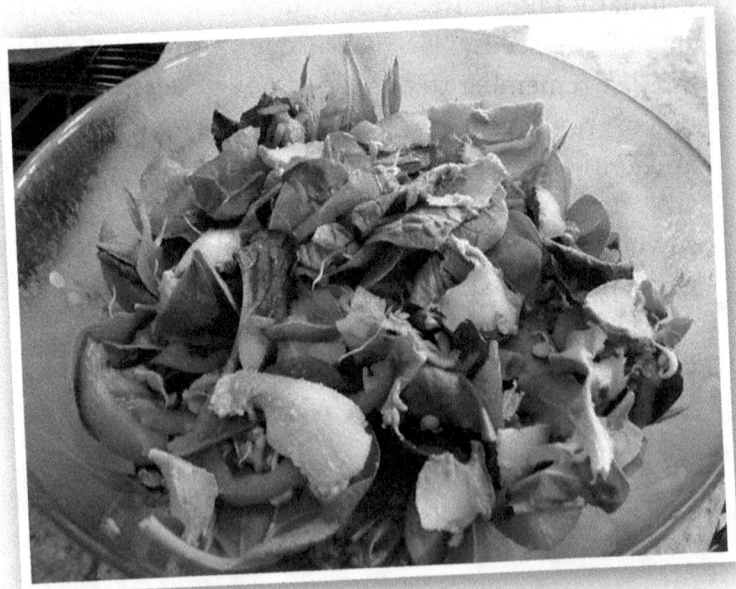

GAEL'S FAVORITE MEALS

For lunch I like to have a large salad with lots of greens, sprouts, grapes, avocado, and veggies. I also have good size pieces of lettuce and put slices of fresh tomatoes and slices of avocados on them and alfalfa sprouts on top. Then I sprinkle with sea salt. Yummy! The salads I eat are very large, so this is actually a filling lunch.

Sometimes I will have a raw veggie burger or a falafel with veggies and sprouts and eat it on dehydrated raw sprouted bread. This way, you can feel like the "other folks" because it is just like a sandwich. These are delicious, and taste much better than they sound. I have a couple of books listed at the end of this book with lots of recipes you can try. If you research on Google in your area, you will be surprised that there just may be some nearby vegan or raw vegan restaurants or cafés that you can try.

I love raw soups with quinoa (a healthy, light grain full of protein and vitamins) and spices in it. I warm the soup in the winter, and eat it cold in the summer. After I warm the soup I throw a big handful of sprouts on top. My favorite soup is tomato. I also like lemon zucchini soup. Soups make a delicious and filling lunch or dinner.

Sometimes I will make a raw pizza using sprouted grains for the crust and raw pizza sauce, and put all kinds of veggies on top. This can be warmed as well or not. I also like to add just a little bit of organic free-range goat cheese, but I keep it separate so that I am aware of how much I'm eating.

SUMMARY

In closing, I want you to remember that healthy eating is not about becoming a vegan or raw vegan like me. You can decide that you will make some changes to the way you eat now by slowly adding bits and pieces of what you have learned, or eliminating or cutting back on some of the foods that are not as good for you. By cutting back on meat eating and dairy, you will benefit tremendously, and by giving up meat and dairy altogether you will see some dramatic health changes for the better. Start adding more organic greens and fruits to your diet and your body will become more vibrant and love you for it. Remember, baby steps, and don't sweat going out to dinner at a friend's home or out at a restaurant. Just do the best you can each day. So what if you don't eat vegetarian or vegan when you go out once in a while? Just go back to the way you usually eat the next day.

This book is especially important in introducing your family to a healthy-eating lifestyle that will benefit them throughout their lives. Like any new dramatic change in your life, it is very easy to get lost and feel like you can't do it alone. After you finish reading this book you will probably lose about 80 percent of what you learned, so use it as a resource to go back to often. It is hard to make a huge change without additional help, which is why I offer coaching services to help get your through the ups and downs of making these changes. I will help you stay on track. There are many other helpful resources on my website, so check it out. If your Company or group would like me to speak, or you know any other company that could benefit from my services, please forward my name and website to them.

My next book will be out this spring of 2012 *The Raw Vegan/Vegan Newbie*, which is a complete step-by-step guide on how to start being a vegan or raw vegan from day one, including how to equip your kitchen, shop, and pack your food for the day.

The summer of 2012 will bring my book, *The Raw Vegan Realtor: Balancing Healthy Eating with a Busy Executive Lifestyle*, which teaches how to avoid the fast food life. This book will be a great resource for all busy executives that are on the road a lot and just can't seem to find the time to eat well.

Check out my web site www.HealthyEating-HealthyBody.com for more services for you, your family, or your company. This site is also a great resource for other books and alternative health choices. Look for my upcoming books listed in the back of this book.

GLOSSARY

acidic: Having a low PH

acetaldehyde: A product of alcohol metabolism that is more toxic than alcohol itself.

alkaline: Having a high PH

aspartame: Also marketed as NutraSweet, Equal, and Amino Sweet, aspartame is a neurotoxin and has been linked to brain cancer, grand mal seizures, and several other central nervous system disorders. This is often found in diet soft drinks.

B12: A vitamin found in organically grown vegetables and animal products. B12 is biosynthesized, which means that it is made by using bacterial enzymes.

BPA (Bisphenol-A): Cancer-causing agent in plastics.

bile: A yellow-green fluid produced by the liver that aids in digestion of fats and the excretion of toxins.

carcinogen: A cancer-causing substance or agent.

casein: The main protein present in dairy. It is used in processed foods and also in adhesives and paints.

chlorophyll: The "blood" of the plant. It is the protein in plant life that gives plants their distinctive green or purple color. When chlorophyll is compared to a molecule of hemoglobin, the oxygen carrier in human blood, it is almost identical. Converts light energy into other forms of energy needed for biochemical processes.

coenzymes: An organic substance that usually contains a vitamin or mineral and combines with a specific protein to form an active enzyme system.

colonic cleanse: Involves the infusion of water into the rectum, called colonic irrigation. This gentle cleansing removes years of old waste and sludge from the intestines, which in turn helps the body repair and take care of itself.

cultured: In the world of food, this is the chemical process of breaking down a complicated substance into simpler parts, usually with the help of bacteria, yeasts, or fungi. Sauerkraut is an example of a cultured vegetable.

DEHA: a carcinogen

enzyme: Any of numerous proteins produced by living organisms and functioning as biochemical catalysts. Found only in raw foods, they work to predigest food in the stomach of a person or animal. They help break down complex food molecules into simpler ones that are acted upon further by the stomach, pancreatic juices, and bile juices until eventually the food is absorbed in the small intestine.

GMO: Means genetically modified. Many of the standard foods we get in the grocery story are genetically modified and have added hormones, which damage our bodies.

mineral: An inorganic element that promotes chemical reactions within the body and is necessary for proper cellular metabolism.

MSG: Monosodium glutamate, which is a food additive used to enhance flavor. Made from glutamic acid; an extitotoxin.

nutrients: Minerals, enzymes, vitamins, oxygen, and proteins.

omega fatty acids: Omega 3, found in fish, fish oils, vegetable oils, and green leafy vegetables; omega 6, found in nuts and grains; omega 9, found in olive oil and avocados.

PH: Potential hydrogen

PH balance: The acid–alkaline balance in our body.

probiotics: "Good bacteria" that live in microbial supplements which improve intestinal balance.

sodium nitrite: A carcinogenic substance used to preserve and color food, especially in meat and fish products.

trans-fats: "Pseudo-fats" produced by the partial hydrogenation of vegetable oils; present in hardened vegetables oils, most margarines, commercial-baked foods, and fried foods; increases the risk of cancer.

tumor: An uncontrolled growth of cells in a specific area; sometimes malignant.

vitamin: An organic substance that acts as a coenzyme or regulator of metabolic processes.

vita mineral greens: Possibly the most healing foods on the planet, and the single most important addition to a diet you can make. Green are a superior, nutritionally dense, therapeutic super-food powder and contains a full spectrum of naturally occurring, absorbable, and non-toxic vitamin, minerals, all the essential amino acids (protein), antioxidants, chlorophyll, soluble and insoluble fibers, tens of thousands of phytonutrients, and a plethora of other synergistically bound, organic nutrients.

whole foods: Foods that are eaten just as they are found in nature.

xenoestrogens: Synthetic estrogens in food.

RECOMMENDED READING

The Hippocrates Diet and Health Program by Ann Wigmore

Healing Cancer from Inside Out by Mike Anderson

Cancer: Step Outside the Box by Ty Bollinger

The Amazing Liver and Gallbladder Flush by Andreas Moritz

Change Your Thoughts, Change Your Life by Dr. Wayne Dyer

BIBLIOGRAPHY

Anderson, Mike. *Healing Cancer from the Inside Out*. United States: RaveDiet.com, 2009.

Bollinger, Ty. *Cancer: Step Outside the Box*. Infinity 510 Squared Partners, 2009.

Campbell, T. Colin, PhD, Thomas M. Campbell II, MD. *The China Study*. Dallas: BenBella, 2006.

Committee on Nutrition and Human Needs. Study: "Dietary Goals for the US." Washington DC: US Government, 1977.

"Composition and Facts about Foods," *Diet Digest*. Mokelumne Hill: Health Research and Raw Food Living, August 16, 2007.

Julius Center for Health Sciences and Primary Care, University Medical Center Utrecht "A High Menaquinone Intake Reduces the Incidence of Coronary Heart Disease." Whole Health Source. March 17, 2009.

Kenner, Robert. *Food Inc*. New York: Magnolia Pictures, 2009. DVD, 93 minutes.

McDougall, John A., MD. "EATING." The McDougall Program, p. 17.

Mirkin, Gabe, MD. "Trans Fats and Type II Diabetes," *Science News.* November 10, 2001, pp. 300–301.

National Research Council Subject. Study: "Diet, Nutrition, and Cancer." Washington DC: National Academy Press, 1982.

Robinson, Jo. *Why Grassfed is Best! The Surprising Benefits of Grassfed Meat, Eggs, and Dairy Products.* Vashon: Vashon Island Press, 2000.

Schachter, Michael B., MD. *HealthWorld*, 2000.

St. Pierre, Brian, CSCS, CISSN. "What They NEVER Want You to Find Out about Real Butter." http://www.getprograde.com/Truth-About-Butter.html. Accessed August 22, 2011.

"Vitamin E, Vitamin A, and Carotene Contents of Alberta Butter." *Journal of Diary Science.* 53(2) pp. 150–154.

Whittaker, Scott, ND. "Colon Health." http://www.tkehealth.com. Accessed August 22, 2011.

ABOUT THE AUTHOR

Gael Dunphy Meyer grew up in Topsfield, Massachusetts. She has been a single parent for the past twenty-six years. Her son Michael Rowan Meyer is an aspiring actor and writer, and the most wonderful thing that has ever happened in Gael's life. Gael grew up in a large family of eight children. She has a driving love for the outdoors, nature, animals, and birds. Gael now resides at her seaside home in Gloucester, Massachusetts. She is known as the "raw vegan realtor" and the "raw vegan speaker"; she has been in real estate for the past twenty-five years. After losing eighty pounds in eight months by changing the way she eats, Gael is now exploring her passion for health in her second life.

Gael is trying to educate people about how simple it really is to regain health and lose weight for good by making smart choices with organic, whole foods. She offers coaching, seminars, and speaking for companies, corporations, and colleges.

She offers Coaching to further maximize results; Seminars for Companies and Corporations, educating employees and employers of the importance of eating right so everyone is more focused, out sick less, and creating a greater performance level; and College Speaking, showing kids the importance of starting now with their eating lifestyle, giving them better health, focus, and energy.

Gael's next book will be out this spring of 2012 *The Raw Vegan/Vegan Newbie*, which is a complete step-by-step guide on how to start being a vegan or raw vegan from day one, including how to equip your kitchen, shop, and pack your food for the day.

The summer of 2012 will bring the next in the series, *The Raw Vegan Realtor: Balancing Healthy Eating with a Busy Executive Lifestyle*, which teaches how to avoid the fast food life. This book will be a great resource for all busy executives that are on the road a lot and just can't seem to find the time to eat well.

For more information on Gael's steps to eating healthy, visit **HealthyEatingHealthyBody.com**, or send Gael an email to:
HealthyEatingHealthyBody@gmail.com

ABOUT HEALTHY EATING HEALTHY BODY

HealthyEatingHealthyBody.com is an easy-to-navigate website where you can find lots of useful information on:

- How Gael lost eighty pounds in eight months (and before and after photos)!

- Gael's weekly blog with lots of fun and helpful banter

- How to obtain coaching from Gael

- Gael's online programs

- Live recorded interviews with other professionals in the field

- How to reach Gael for your future seminars

- Updated articles relating to Healthy Eating

- Recommended reading in related topics

- Gael's favorite weekly recipes

- Gael's affiliate programs

- Gael's books and products
- Your comments and suggestions

For more information on Gael's steps to eating healthy, visit HealthyEatingHealthyBody.com, or send Gael an email to:

HealthyEatingHealthyBody@gmail.com